FITNESS FOOD

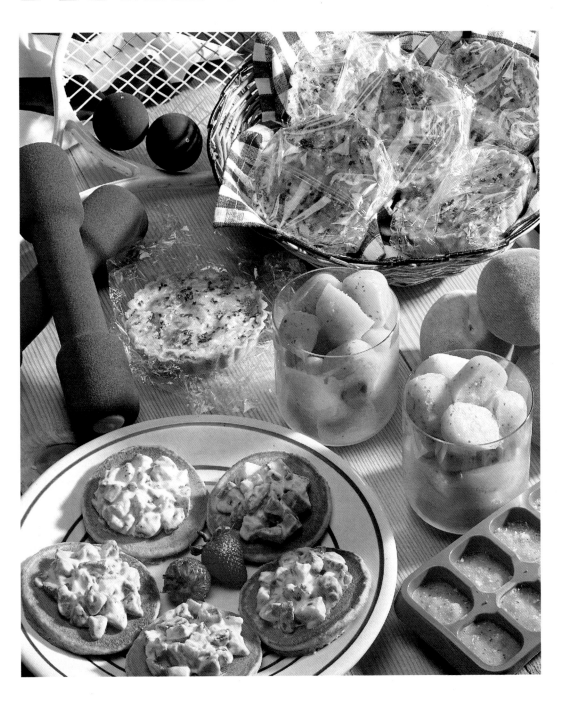

UK COOKERY EDITOR
Robyn Ayrdon

EDITORIAL
Text: Helen O'Connor B Sc Dip N.D.
Food Editor: Sheryle Eastwood
Assistant Food Editor: Anneka Mitchell
Home Economist: Donna Hay
Recipe Development: Belinda Clayton,
Sue Geraghty
Editorial Coordinator: Margaret Kelly

PHOTOGRAPHY
Harm Mol

STYLING
Wendy Berecry

DESIGN AND PRODUCTION
Manager: Nadia Sbisa
Senior Production Editor:
Rachel Blackmore
Layout: Claire Pallant
Finished Art: Chris Hatcher
Cover Design: Frank Pithers

PUBLISHER
Philippa Sandall

JBFP 103 UK
Includes Index
ISBN 1 86343 0342

Published by J.B. Fairfax Press Pty Limited
A.C.N. 003 738 430
Formatted by J.B. Fairfax Press Pty Limited
Output by Adtype, Sydney
Printed by Toppan Printing Co, Singapore

Distributed by J.B. Fairfax Press Ltd
9 Trinity Centre, Park Farm Estate
Wellingborough, Northants, UK
Ph: (0933) 402330 Fax: (0933) 402234

NUTRITIONAL DATA
Tables on pages 13, 36, 52 and 53
'This work is the copyright of the
Commonwealth of Australia and includes
some copyright nutrient composition data
provided by Associate Professor H.
Greenfield, Professor R.B.H. Wills and others at the University of New South Wales. All
these data are reproduced by
permission.'

Contents

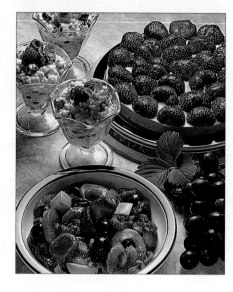

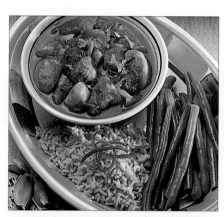

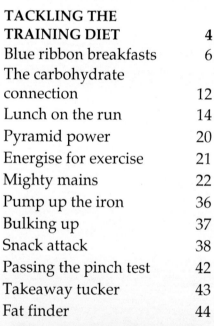

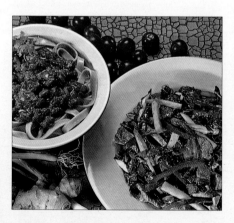

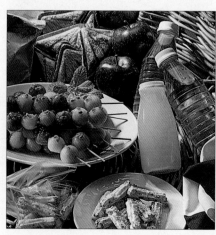

Foreword

Even in the early days of my athletic career I considered nutrition to be an important part of my lifestyle. My goals have been not only to enjoy food and to eat a healthy diet, but to attend to the special nutritional needs of my sport. Over the last ten years I have been excited to watch the increase in knowledge and interest in the specialised field of diet for athletic performance.

While scientists can now advise us on many principles of sports nutrition – for example, eating for recovery, loading up for competition day, and looking after increased iron requirements – sportspeople need help to turn the theories and knowledge into food for the table. This book Fitness Food *is a welcome addition to the sportsperson's library – and kitchen.*

With clear and up-to-date information on many areas of nutrition for sportspeople, it presents a great overview of the issues that we may face in our sport or exercise. More than this, it provides simple and enjoyable ways of putting this advice into practice. What you eat can make a difference to the way you perform. Fitness Food *can help you achieve the best from your food and the best in your sport, whatever your goals.*

Robert de Castella
Olympic and Commonwealth
Marathon Runner

ABOUT THIS BOOK

Nutritional analysis: Each recipe has been computer analysed for its calorie (kilojoule) content and nutrient value. At a glance, you can see how much protein a dish contains and whether it is LOW, MEDIUM or HIGH in carbohydrate, fat and fibre. The following guidelines have been used.

Carbohydrate (% energy):
    less than 50% .... Low
    50-60%   .... Medium
    greater than 60% .... High
Fat (% energy):
    less than 20% .... Low
    20-35%   .... Medium
    greater than 35% .... High
Fibre:
    less than 2 g per serve .... Low
    2-6 g per serve .... Medium
    greater than 6 g per serve ..... High

Microwave: Where microwave instructions occur in this book a microwave oven with a 650 watt output has been used. Wattage on domestic microwave ovens varies between 500 and 700 watts, and it may be necessary to vary cooking times slightly depending on your oven.

Check-and-Go: Use the easy Check-and-Go boxes which appear beside each ingredient. Simply check your pantry and if the ingredients are not there, tick the boxes as a reminder to add those items to your shopping list.

Canned foods: Can sizes vary between countries and manufacturers. You may find the quantities in this book are slightly different from what is available in your supermarket. Purchase the can nearest to the size suggested in the recipe.

Symbols: The recipes in this book have been marked with the following symbols.

Takes less than 15 minutes

Takes less than 30 minutes

Takes 45 minutes or longer

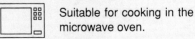

Suitable for cooking in the microwave oven.

Suitable for people on a vegetarian diet

Tackling the training diet

Regardless of the sport you play or your fitness and exercise program, the basic dietary principles are similar. The right quality and quantity of food helps active people perform at their best.

DIET CHECKLIST

Balance: A well balanced diet is essential for good health and is the basis of peak performance.

Eat regularly: Active people in heavy training need to eat regularly to ensure that they refuel their bodies for the strenuous training sessions ahead. Nutritious snacks are usually required also to top up energy levels through the day. Those who skip meals often fail to consume adequate amounts of energy, carbohydrate, fluid and other essential nutrients.

Energy: The energy content of your diet is related to how much fuel you use each day. The more active you are, the more fuel you require. Energy needs are measured in calories (kilojoules). Balancing the energy you eat with the energy you use is essential for peak performance. Inadequate energy will result in fatigue and weight loss; excess energy will lead to weight gain.

Carbohydrate: To perform at its best the body requires the right type of fuel. No matter what your sport, carbohydrates are the best type of fuel for you! High carbohydrate diets help to enhance stamina and prevent fatigue. Complex carbohydrate (starch), which includes breakfast cereals, bread, pasta, rice and potatoes, should provide the majority of the carbohydrate eaten. Simple carbohydrate – sugar, honey, confectionery and soft drinks – should provide less than 15 per cent of your daily energy.

Fluids: The human body is 60 per cent water. During exercise some of this water is lost as sweat, and extra fluid must be consumed to replace it. If these losses are not replaced, dehydration occurs and the body overheats – just like a car without a radiator! Mild dehydration decreases athletic performance by reducing strength and stamina: severe dehydration can be life threatening. In most cases, cool water is the best fluid replacement drink.

Alcohol: While alcohol offers no benefit to athletic performance, a moderate alcohol intake is unlikely to be detrimental – providing it does not exceed 'safe limits' and is not taken close to the time of competition.

Salt: Although sweat contains salt, the amount of salt lost in training is easily replaced by a well balanced diet – even without adding salt to food. Training also results in adaptations which improve the body's ability to conserve salt. The salt content of sweat is less in well-trained athletes. Since high-salt diets in-

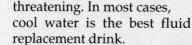
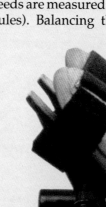

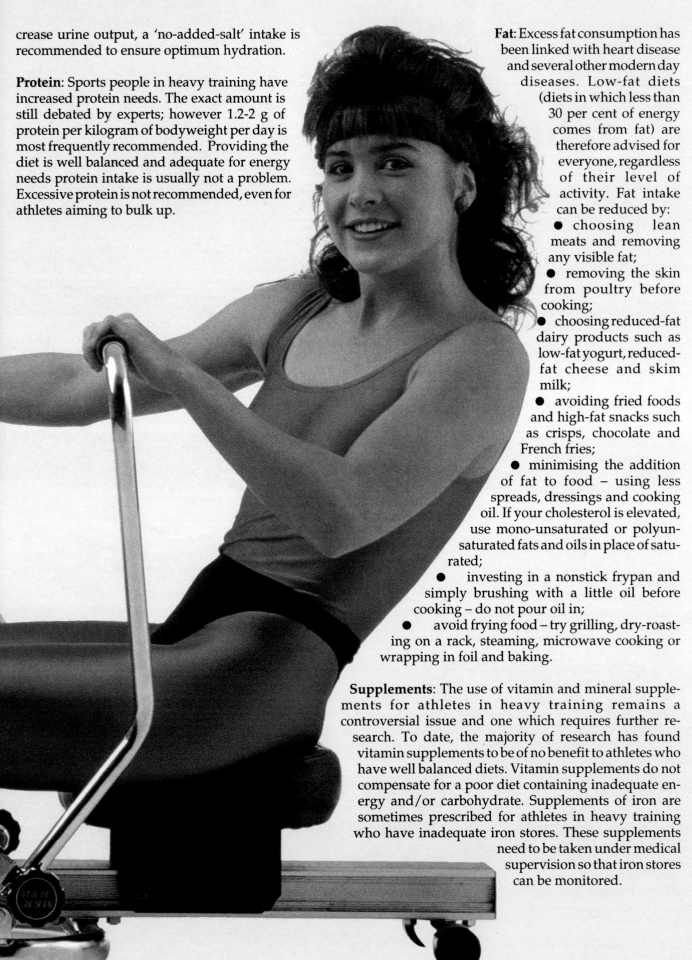

crease urine output, a 'no-added-salt' intake is recommended to ensure optimum hydration.

Protein: Sports people in heavy training have increased protein needs. The exact amount is still debated by experts; however 1.2-2 g of protein per kilogram of bodyweight per day is most frequently recommended. Providing the diet is well balanced and adequate for energy needs protein intake is usually not a problem. Excessive protein is not recommended, even for athletes aiming to bulk up.

Fat: Excess fat consumption has been linked with heart disease and several other modern day diseases. Low-fat diets (diets in which less than 30 per cent of energy comes from fat) are therefore advised for everyone, regardless of their level of activity. Fat intake can be reduced by:

- choosing lean meats and removing any visible fat;
- removing the skin from poultry before cooking;
- choosing reduced-fat dairy products such as low-fat yogurt, reduced-fat cheese and skim milk;
- avoiding fried foods and high-fat snacks such as crisps, chocolate and French fries;
- minimising the addition of fat to food – using less spreads, dressings and cooking oil. If your cholesterol is elevated, use mono-unsaturated or polyunsaturated fats and oils in place of saturated;
- investing in a nonstick frypan and simply brushing with a little oil before cooking – do not pour oil in;
- avoid frying food – try grilling, dry-roasting on a rack, steaming, microwave cooking or wrapping in foil and baking.

Supplements: The use of vitamin and mineral supplements for athletes in heavy training remains a controversial issue and one which requires further research. To date, the majority of research has found vitamin supplements to be of no benefit to athletes who have well balanced diets. Vitamin supplements do not compensate for a poor diet containing inadequate energy and/or carbohydrate. Supplements of iron are sometimes prescribed for athletes in heavy training who have inadequate iron stores. These supplements need to be taken under medical supervision so that iron stores can be monitored.

Blue ribbon breakfasts

MIGHTY MUESLI

Makes 20 servings
Oven temperature 180°C, 350°, Gas 4

 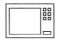

- ☐ **375 g (12 oz) rolled oats**
- ☐ **2 tablespoons shredded coconut**
- ☐ **3 tablespoons oat bran**
- ☐ **3 tablespoons wheat germ**
- ☐ **45 g (1¹/₂ oz) oat flakes**
- ☐ **3 tablespoons sunflower seeds**
- ☐ **4 tablespoons chopped dried peaches**
- ☐ **3 tablespoons chopped dried pears**
- ☐ **3 tablespoons currants**

1 Place rolled oats and coconut in a baking dish and bake for 15-20 minutes, or until oats and coconut are toasted. Stir several times during cooking to ensure even toasting. Remove from oven and set aside to cool.

2 Place cooled rolled oats and coconut, oat bran, wheat germ, oat flakes, sunflower seeds, dried peaches, dried pears and currants in a bowl. Mix well to combine.

Serving suggestion: Sprinkle with banana chips if desired and top with ice cold milk or fruit juice.

To microwave: The rolled oats and coconut can be toasted in minutes in the microwave. To toast rolled oats, place in a microwave-safe ceramic or glass dish and cook on HIGH (100%), stirring every 2 minutes for 5-6 minutes, or until rolled oats are golden and crisp. To toast coconut, place in a microwave-safe ceramic or glass dish and cook on HIGH (100%), stirring every minute, for 2-3 minutes or until toasted. The length of time the coconut takes to toast will vary depending on the amount of moisture in it, so watch carefully as it will burn easily.

To store: Place in an airtight container and keep on hand for a quick and filling breakfast.

125 Calories (530 kilojoules) per serve
Carbohydrate	20.0 g	High
Protein	4.0 g	
Fat	3.0 g	Medium
Fibre	3.8 g	Medium

SPICY PANCAKES

Serves 4

- ☐ **3 tablespoons buckwheat flour, sifted**
- ☐ **3 tablespoons self-raising flour, sifted**
- ☐ **1 teaspoon ground allspice**
- ☐ **1 tablespoon honey, warmed**
- ☐ **250 mL (8 fl oz) skimmed milk**
- ☐ **1 teaspoon vegetable oil**
- ☐ **1 egg white, lightly beaten**
- ☐ **1 teaspoon grated lemon rind**

1 Place buckwheat and self-raising flours with allspice in a mixing bowl. Combine honey, skim milk, oil and egg white. Stir into flour mixture and mix to a smooth batter. Mix in lemon rind.

2 Drop tablespoons of mixture into a heated nonstick frying pan and cook until golden on both sides.

Serving suggestion: Top pancakes with Banana Yogurt Topping or Berry Sauce. These pancakes are also delicious served plain.

135 Calories (565 kilojoules) per serve
Carbohydrate	24.0 g	High
Protein	6.0 g	
Fat	2.0 g	Low
Fibre	1.2 g	Low

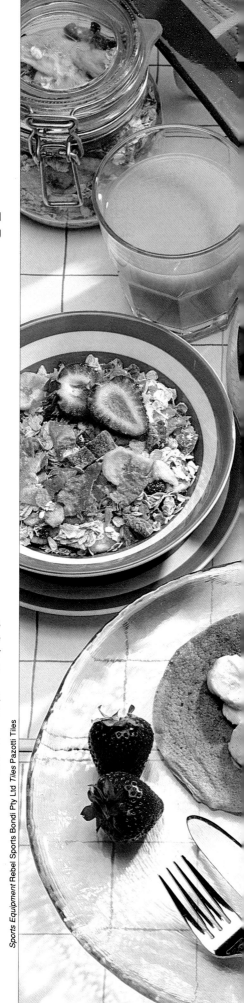

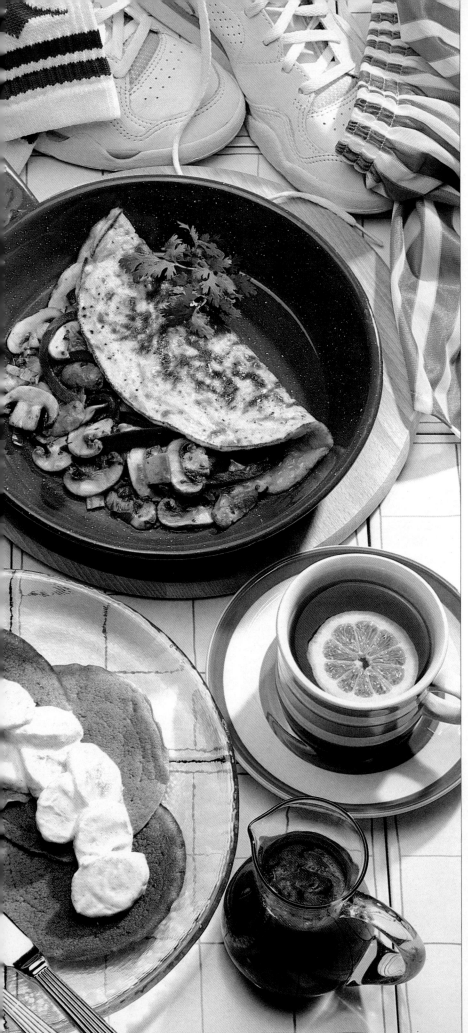

BANANA YOGURT TOPPING

Makes 250 g (8 oz)

☐ **1 banana, sliced**
☐ **185 g (6 oz) low-fat natural yogurt**
☐ **¹/₂ teaspoon ground cinnamon**

Place banana, yogurt and cinnamon in a bowl and mix well.
Serving suggestion: Use as a topping for pancakes, or spoon over cereal or fruit.

30 Calories (120 kilojoules) per serve		
Carbohydrate	5.0 g	High
Protein	1.5 g	
Fat	neg	Low
Fibre	neg	Low

BERRY SAUCE

Makes 250 mL (8 fl oz)

☐ **250 g (8 oz) mixed berries, fresh or frozen**
☐ **2 tablespoons apple juice**

Place berries in a food processor or blender and process until smooth. Strain through a sieve to remove seeds, and stir in apple juice.
Serving suggestion: Spoon over pancakes, cereal or fruit.

15 Calories (55 kilojoules) per serve		
Carbohydrate	3.0 g	High
Protein	neg	
Fat	neg	Low
Fibre	neg	Low

Spring Omelette (page 8), Berry Sauce, Spicy Pancakes with Banana Yogurt Topping, Mighty Muesli

SPRING OMELETTE

Serves 2

- ☐ 1 teaspoon polyunsaturated margarine
- ☐ 4 eggs, lightly beaten
- ☐ 3 tablespoons skimmed milk
- ☐ freshly ground black pepper
- ☐ 3 tablespoons grated reduced-fat cheddar cheese

VEGETABLE FILLING
- ☐ 1 teaspoon polyunsaturated margarine
- ☐ 2 spring onions, finely chopped
- ☐ 6 button mushrooms, sliced
- ☐ ½ small red pepper, sliced
- ☐ 1 teaspoon chopped fresh coriander

1 To make filling, melt margarine in a nonstick frying pan and cook spring onions, mushrooms, red pepper and coriander over a low heat for 2 minutes or until tender. Remove vegetables from pan, set aside and keep warm.

2 Melt margarine in a clean nonstick frying pan. Combine eggs, milk and black pepper to taste in bowl. Pour into pan and cook over a low heat until almost set. Top half the omelette with filling, then sprinkle with cheese. Fold omelette over, cut into half, slide onto serving plates and serve immediately.

Serving suggestion: Start your breakfast with fresh fruit then serve the omelette with crisp toast.

135 Calories (570 kilojoules) per serve

Carbohydrate	*1.5 g*	*Low*
Protein	*10.0 g*	
Fat	*10.0 g*	*High*
Fibre	*0.5 g*	*Low*

PEACHES AND CREAM MUFFINS

Serves 2

- ☐ 2 muffins, halved and toasted

PEACHES AND CREAM TOPPING
- ☐ 4 tablespoons low-fat cottage cheese
- ☐ pulp of 1 passion fruit
- ☐ 2 peaches, stoned and sliced

Combine cottage cheese and passion fruit pulp in a bowl. Spread mixture over muffin halves, top with peach slices and serve.

225 Calories (950 kilojoules) per serve

Carbohydrate	*37.0 g*	*High*
Protein	*14.0 g*	
Fat	*2.0 g*	*Low*
Fibre	*4.8 g*	*Medium*

FRUIT AND NUT MUFFINS

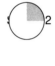2

- ☐ 2 muffins, halved and toasted

FRUIT AND NUT TOPPING
- ☐ 4 tablespoons low-fat cottage cheese
- ☐ 1 tablespoon currants
- ☐ 1 tablespoon chopped raisins
- ☐ 1 teaspoon grated orange rind
- ☐ 2 tablespoons chopped pecan nuts or walnuts

Place ricotta cheese, currants, raisins and orange rind in a bowl. Mix to combine and spread over muffin halves. Sprinkle with pecan nuts and serve.

Hint: Use wholemeal or mixed grain muffins to increase your fibre intake.

295 Calories (1240 kilojoules) per serve

Carbohydrate	*40.0 g*	*Medium*
Protein	*12.0 g*	
Fat	*10.0 g*	*Medium*
Fibre	*3.3 g*	*Medium*

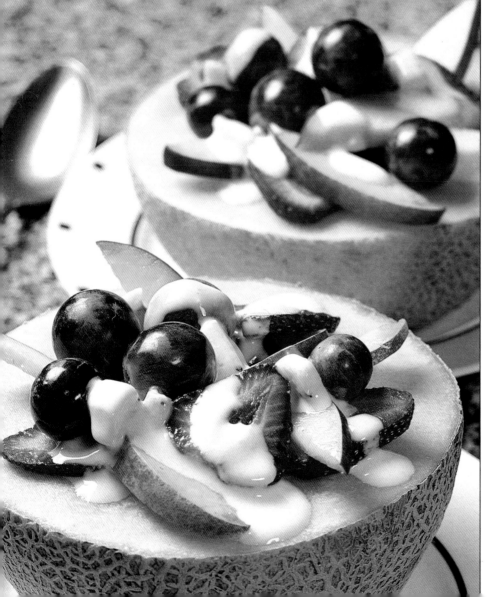

Melon Cups with Yogurt Dressing

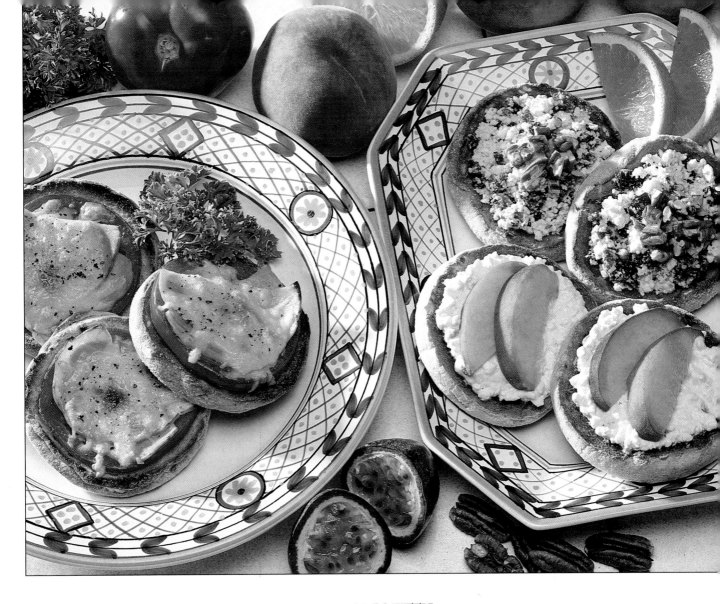

TURKEY MUFFINS

Serves 2

☐ **2 muffins, halved and toasted**

TOPPING
☐ **1 tomato, sliced**
☐ **2 slices cooked turkey breast**
☐ **3 tablespoons grated low-fat cheddar cheese**
☐ **freshly ground black pepper**

Place tomato slices on muffin halves. Top with turkey slices, cheese and black pepper to taste. Place under a preheated grill until heated through.

250 Calories (1055 kilojoules) per serve

Carbohydrate	31.0 g	Medium
Protein	22.0 g	
Fat	4.0 g	Low
Fibre	2.5 g	Medium

MELON CUPS WITH YOGURT DRESSING

Serves 4

☐ **2 small melons such as charentais, galia or ogen, halved and seeds removed**
☐ **2 nectarines, stones removed and sliced**
☐ **155 g (5 oz) strawberries, hulled and sliced**
☐ **155 g (5 oz) black grapes**

YOGURT DRESSING
☐ **185 g (6 oz) low-fat natural yogurt**
☐ **1 tablespoon honey**
☐ **1 kiwi fruit, peeled and roughly chopped**

1 To make dressing, place yogurt, honey and kiwi fruit in a bowl and mix to combine.
2 Place melon halves on individual serving plates. Fill with nectarines, strawberries and grapes. Spoon dressing over fruit in melon halves and chill.
Serving suggestion: Start your breakfast with a milk drink and finish with bread or toast.

155 Calories (650 kilojoules) per serve

Carbohydrate	32.0 g	High
Protein	5.0 g	
Fat	neg g	Low
Fibre	5.0 g	Medium

Turkey Muffins, Fruit and Nut Muffins, Peaches and Cream Muffins

FRUITY PORRIDGE

Serves 2

- ☐ 3 tablespoons chopped dried apricots
- ☐ 1 small apple, cored and chopped
- ☐ 125 mL (4 fl oz) water
- ☐ 500 mL (16 fl oz) skimmed milk
- ☐ 315 g (10 oz) instant rolled oats
- ☐ 1 teaspoon mixed spice
- ☐ 2 tablespoons sultanas

1 Place apricots, apple and water in a saucepan. Bring to the boil, then reduce heat and simmer for 5 minutes or until fruit is tender.
2 Place milk in a saucepan and heat gently for 2-3 minutes. Stir in rolled oats, bring to the boil and cook, stirring constantly, for 1 minute. Stir in apricots, apple, mixed spice and sultanas.
Serving suggestion: Top with extra skimmed milk and sprinkle with grated nutmeg.
To microwave: Place apricots, apple and water in a large 2 litre (3$\frac{1}{2}$ pt) microwave-safe bowl or jug and cook on HIGH (100%) for 2-3 minutes, or until fruit is soft. Heat milk on HIGH (100%) for 1 minute, stir in rolled oats and cook for 1 minute. Stir once during cooking. Mix in apricots, apple, mixed spice and sultanas.

490 Calories (2050 kilojoules) per serve

Carbohydrate	88.0 g	High
Protein	19.0 g	
Fat	6.0 g	Low
Fibre	14.2 g	High

CALORIE SAVER

The unsweetened varieties of canned fruit and fruit juice will cut calories (kilojoules) without affecting the recipe, so are a good alternative for those watching their weight.

CARBOHYDRATE CHARGES

Top ready-made cereals with any of the following to add extra energy, carbohydrate or fibre:
- ● Dried fruit, such as sultanas, raisins, dates, apricots or figs.
- ● Mashed or sliced bananas.
- ● Stewed or canned fruits, such as apples, pears, peaches or pineapples.
- ● A drizzle of honey or a sprinkle of sugar.
- ● Chopped nuts.
- ● A sprinkle of sesame, sunflower or pumpkin seeds.
- ● A spoonful of wheat germ, lecithin or bran.
- ● Low-fat yogurt for extra calcium.
- ● Fortified milk for extra calcium, protein and energy.

VEGETABLE HASH BROWNS

Serves 4

- ☐ 2 potatoes, peeled and grated
- ☐ 1 carrot, peeled and grated
- ☐ 1 courgette, grated
- ☐ 1 tablespoon poppy seeds
- ☐ 2 eggs, lightly beaten
- ☐ freshly ground black pepper
- ☐ 1 tablespoon polyunsaturated vegetable oil

1 Place potatoes, carrot, courgette, poppy seeds and eggs in a bowl. Season to taste with black pepper and mix well to combine.
2 Brush a nonstick frying pan with oil and heat. Place spoonfuls of mixture in pan and flatten slightly. Cook for 4-5 minutes each side or until golden.
Serving suggestion: For a complete breakfast, start with a glass of skim milk – or one of the drinks from Dive into a Drink (see page 50) – fruit, and serve the hash browns with bread or toast.

120 Calories (500 kilojoules) per serve

Carbohydrate	9.0 g	Low
Protein	5.0 g	
Fat	7.0 g	High
Fibre	2.2 g	Medium

TASTY HAWAIIAN POCKETS

Serves 4
Oven temperature 180°C, 350°F, Gas 4

- ☐ 4 small wholemeal pitta breads

HAWAIIAN FILLING
- ☐ 125 g (4 oz) low-fat cottage cheese
- ☐ 3 tablespoons grated low-fat cheddar cheese
- ☐ 220 g (7 oz) canned pineapple pieces, chopped
- ☐ 4 slices lean ham, finely chopped
- ☐ 1 tablespoon snipped chives
- ☐ freshly ground black pepper
- ☐ 1 teaspoon polyunsaturated oil

1 To make filling, place cottage cheese, cheddar cheese, pineapple and ham in a bowl. Season to taste with black pepper and mix to combine.
2 Make a small slit in the side of each pitta bread and spoon in filling. Brush a nonstick frying pan with oil and heat over a medium heat. Cook pockets for 3 minutes each side or until crisp and heated through.
Serving suggestion: Accompany with a fruit smoothie (see page 50).

335 Calories (1415 kilojoules) per serve

Carbohydrate	52.0 g	High
Protein	21.0 g	
Fat	5.0 g	Low
Fibre	4.7 g	Medium

Vegetable Hash Browns, Fruity Porridge, Tasty Hawaiian Pockets

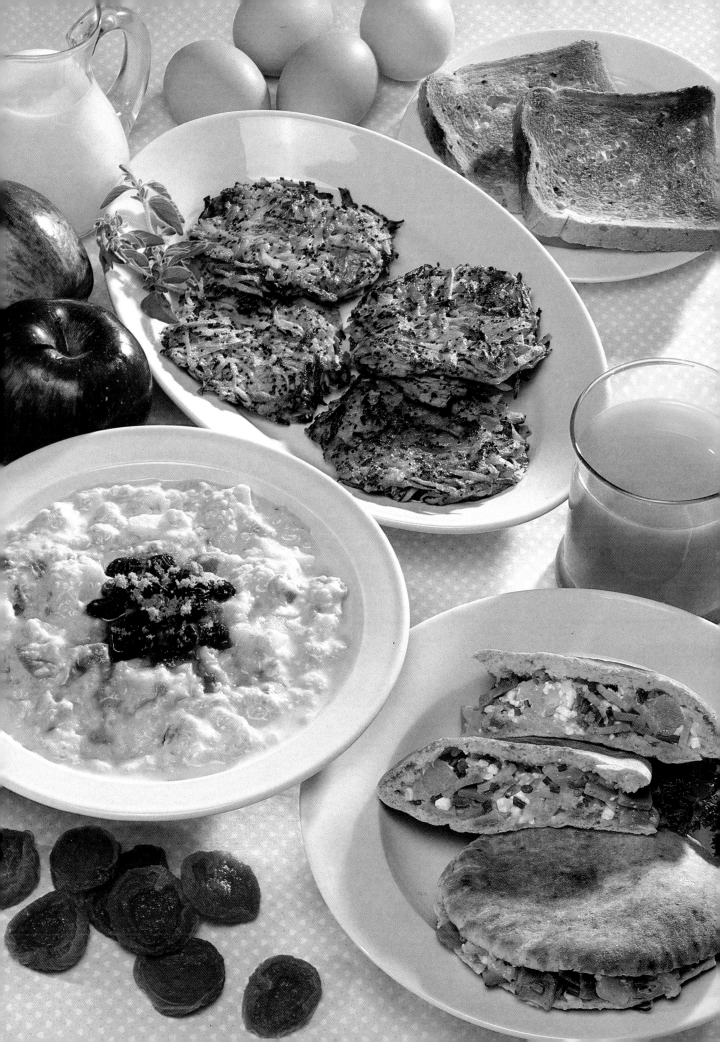

The carbohydrate connection

CARBO CALCULATOR

Normal daily carbohydrate requirements are:
4.5 grams carbohydrate per kilogram of bodyweight.
Daily carbohydrate requirements for endurance/heavy training are:
8-10 grams carbohydrate per kilogram of bodyweight.

Boiled brown rice
180 g
57 g carbohydrate
1.6 g fibre

Banana
1 medium
30 g carbohydrate
3.7 g fibre

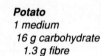

Baked beans
1 cup (165 g)
16 g carbohydrate
12 g fibre

Potato
1 medium
16 g carbohydrate
1.3 g fibre

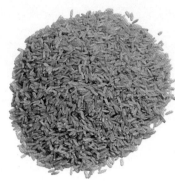

Cooked rolled oats
260 g cooked
22 g carbohydrate
3.4 g fibre

White bread
1 slice
13 g carbohydrate
0.8 g fibre

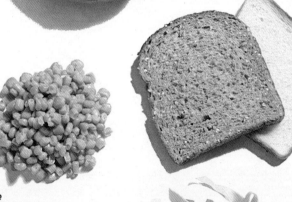

Mixed grain bread
1 slice
12 g carbohydrate
1.4 g fibre

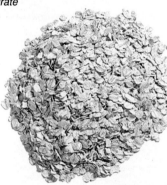

Apple
1 medium
18 g carbohydrate
3 g fibre

Sweet corn
80 g
20 g carbohydrate
3.5 g fibre

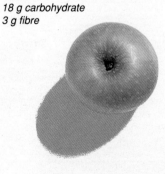

Muesli (untoasted)
62 g
33 g carbohydrate
7.8 g fibre

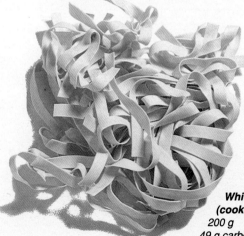

White pasta (cooked)
200 g
49 g carbohydrate
3.6 g fibre

Carbohydrate is stored in the body as glucose in the blood (blood sugar), and as glycogen in the liver and muscles.

Glycogen, made up of units of glucose, is an important source of energy for active people. When glycogen stores are depleted, fatigue sets in and performance suffers. The amount of glycogen required depends on the duration, type and intensity of exercise.

To maintain adequate glycogen stores for training, active people should aim to consume 55-60 per cent of their energy requirements as carbohydrate. Endurance athletes need to aim for about 70 per cent.

Complex carbohydrate (starch) should make up most of the carbohydrate consumed. It sustains blood sugar levels more effectively than simple carbohydrate (sugars). Complex carbohydrate foods are also a better source of vitamins, minerals and fibre.
Sources: bread, breakfast cereal, rice, pasta, potato, dried peas and beans, etc.

Simple carbohydrate should supply less than 15 per cent of the total carbohydrate intake.
Sources: sugar, honey, jam, confectionery, soft drinks, etc.

Carbohydrate (glycogen) loading: Increasing or 'loading' glycogen stores is important for athletes taking part in endurance competitions which involve greater than 90 minutes of strenuous, uninterrupted effort. The 'extra' glycogen store helps to delay fatigue and enhance staying power. Glycogen loading also helps to prevent hypoglycaemia – low blood sugar.

In sports where speed, agility and flexibility are more important than stamina the extra weight of glycogen and the water that is stored with it (3 grams for each gram of glycogen), is likely to be detrimental. An adequate, rather than 'loaded' store is appropriate

for these sports.

Loading up:
● Commence carbohydrate loading 3-4 days prior to competition.
● Increase carbohydrate intake to 70-85 per cent of energy (about 8-10 grams of carbohydrate per kilogram (pound) of bodyweight).
● Decrease training to reduce the use of muscle glycogen.

HYPOGLYCAEMIA

Endurance exercise can reduce blood sugar and glycogen stores to dangerously low levels. A low blood sugar level – hypoglycaemia – can cause symptoms such as dizziness, shakiness, faintness and confusion. In severe cases there is also risk of collapse.

● Sports such as marathons, triathlons and iron-man events require high levels of endurance.
● Other sports, like shot put, high jump and sprint events are based on repeated, short periods of non-endurance exercise.
● The vast majority of sports fall somewhere between these two extremes.
● The longer the duration of strenuous, uninterrupted effort the greater the endurance required.

CARBOHYDRATE COUNTER

FOOD	SERVE SIZE	CARBOHYDRATE (g)
BREAD		
Wholemeal bread	1 slice	11
Raisin bread	1 slice	17
Lebanese bread	1 round	57
Wholemeal crispbread	2 biscuits	8
CEREALS		
Cornflakes	30 g (1 oz)	25
Muesli (untoasted)	60 g (2 oz)	33
Rolled oats (cooked)	250 g (8 oz)	22
FRUIT		
Orange	1 medium	12
Orange juice	250 mL (8 fl oz)	20
Pear	1 medium	19
Rockmelon	155 g (5 oz)	8
Sultanas	1 tablespoon	9
PASTA AND RICE (cooked)		
Egg pasta	200 g	51
Spinach pasta	200 g	55
Wholemeal pasta	200 g	49
Brown rice	185 g (6 oz)	57
White rice	185 g (6 oz)	53
VEGETABLES AND LEGUMES		
Cooked lentils	170 g (5½ oz)	26
Potato	1 medium	16

Lunch on the run

GOLDEN GRAIN SALAD

Serves 4

- ☐ 220 g (7 oz) brown rice, cooked
- ☐ 220 g (7 oz) pearl barley, cooked
- ☐ 60 g (2 oz) couscous, cooked
- ☐ 440 g (14 oz) canned sweet corn kernels, no-added-salt, drained
- ☐ 1 green pepper, cut into strips
- ☐ 1 carrot, peeled and cut into strips
- ☐ 2 stalks celery, cut into strips
- ☐ 1 courgette, cut into strips

ORANGE DRESSING
- ☐ 125 mL (4 fl oz) orange juice
- ☐ 2 teaspoons wholegrain mustard
- ☐ 1 teaspoon finely grated fresh ginger
- ☐ freshly ground black pepper

1   Place rice, barley, couscous, sweet corn, green pepper, carrot, celery and courgette in a large serving bowl.
2   To make dressing, place orange juice, mustard, ginger, and black pepper to taste in a screwtop jar. Shake well to combine. Pour over salad and toss to combine.
Do ahead: Keep a selection of cooked rice, pasta and legumes in the refrigerator then you will always have carbohydrate-rich food that can be made into a salad in minutes. Always cook extra of these foods to have on hand.

620 Calories (2590 kilojoules) per serve

Carbohydrate	127.0 g	High
Protein	14.0 g	
Fat	5.0 g	Low
Fibre	11.0 g	High

CHICKEN PASTA ROLLS

Serves 4

- ☐ 12 spinach or wholemeal lasagne sheets
- ☐ 2 tablespoons grated fresh Parmesan cheese

CHICKEN AND LEEK FILLING
- ☐ 2 teaspoons polyunsaturated oil
- ☐ 3 leeks, washed, finely sliced
- ☐ 3 chicken breast fillets, cut into thin strips
- ☐ 125 mL (4 fl oz) chicken stock
- ☐ 3 teaspoons cornflour blended with 2 tablespoons of water
- ☐ 1 teaspoon French mustard
- ☐ 2 tablespoons chopped fresh basil

1   Cook lasagne sheets in boiling water in a large saucepan until tender. Drain and set aside to keep warm.
2   To make filling, heat oil in a large frying pan and cook leeks and chicken, for 4-5 minutes or until brown. Stir in stock, cornflour mixture, mustard and basil and cook, stirring, for 2 minutes longer.
3   Place spoonfuls of filling on pasta sheets, roll up, top with Parmesan cheese and serve immediately.
Serving suggestion: For extra fibre and carbohydrate serve with a green salad and crusty wholemeal bread.

285 Calories (1200 kilojoules) per serve

Carbohydrate	28.0 g	Low
Protein	25.0 g	
Fat	8.0 g	Medium
Fibre	3.1 g	Medium

Multi-Layered Bread Loaf, Golden Grain Salad, Chicken Pasta Rolls

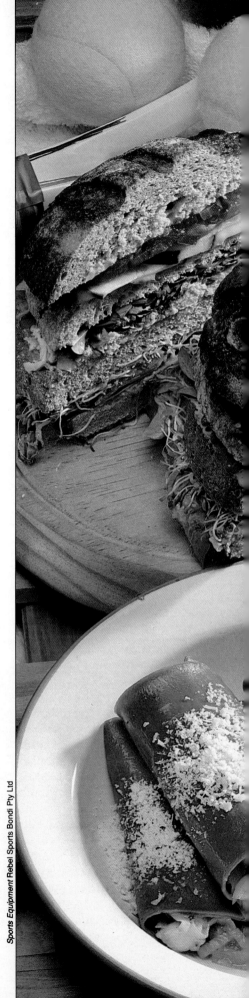

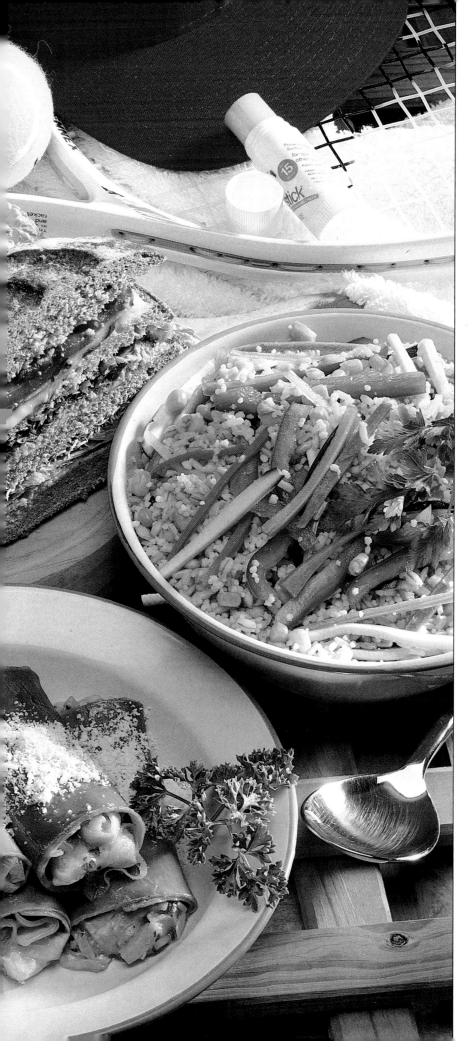

MULTI-LAYERED BREAD LOAF

Serves 2

- ☐ **1 small round rye cottage loaf**
- ☐ **2 tablespoons reduced-fat mayonnaise**
- ☐ **1 tablespoon wholegrain mustard**
- ☐ **4 cos lettuce leaves**
- ☐ **4 oak leaf lettuce leaves**
- ☐ **30 g (1 oz) alfalfa sprouts**
- ☐ **105 g (3^1/$_2$ oz) canned pink salmon, no-added-salt, drained**
- ☐ **2 spring onions, finely chopped**
- ☐ **30 g (1 oz) watercress**
- ☐ **2 tomatoes, sliced**
- ☐ **^{1}/$_2$ cucumber, sliced**
- ☐ **1 tablespoon freshly chopped basil**
- ☐ **freshly ground black pepper**

1 Cut bread horizontally into four even layers. Place mayonnaise and mustard in a small bowl and mix to combine. Spread each bread layer with mayonnaise mixture.
2 Arrange cos and oak leaf lettuce leaves and sprouts over bottom layer of bread. Top with next bread layer. Then spread with salmon and top with spring onions and watercress. Top with next bread round, then arrange tomato and cucumber slices over bread round, sprinkle with basil and black pepper to taste. Finally top with remaining bread round.

Serving suggestion: Cut into wedges to serve and accompany with fresh fruit.

Variation: This multi-layered sandwich could also be made using individual bread rolls. Choose four large bread rolls in place of the cottage loaf. Cut each roll horizontally into four even layers and assemble as described above, remembering to divide the ingredients evenly between each roll.

710 Calories (2965 kilojoules) per serve

Carbohydrate	*108.0 g*	*High*
Protein	*32.0 g*	
Fat	*14.0 g*	*Low*
Fibre	*11.0 g*	*High*

SUPER 'SAND-WEDGES'

Sandwiches remain the most popular and convenient lunch for people 'on the go'. Changing the type of bread and filling helps to prevent boredom. Try some of the following ideas and remember to use as little margarine or butter as possible – better still, leave it off altogether.

SERVING SUGGESTIONS

Tri-wedges: Include a third piece of bread in the centre of the sandwich – it adds extra carbohydrate and is just as quick to eat.

Toast-wedges: When you feel like something hot, toast your sandwich under a grill, or cook it in a sandwich maker. Preheat the grill or sandwich maker while you are making the sandwich.

Pocket-wedges: Place filling in a pitta bread.

Roll-wedges: Place fillings on naan or pitta bread and roll up. One large round is equivalent to four slices of bread.

Continental-wedges: Try some of the different breads and rolls that are now available such as rye, black, pumpernickel or bagels.

Crisp-wedges: Top crispbread or rice cakes with fillings of your choice.

FILLING IDEAS

● Lean roast meat with pickle, mustard or chutney and lettuce, tomato or mixed salad.

● Cooked chicken or turkey (skin removed) with reduced-fat mayonnaise or cranberry sauce and lettuce, mixed salad, avocado, celery, sprouts or chopped walnuts.

● Cheese (reduced-fat-and-salt varieties) with celery, lettuce, mixed salad, grated carrot and sultanas, canned or fresh pineapple slices, leam ham, or gherkin.

● Cottage or ricotta cheese with dried fruit, chopped walnuts, pine nuts, lettuce, mixed salad, tomato, grated carrot and sultanas, chopped dried dates, whole grain mustard, hummus, or tahini.

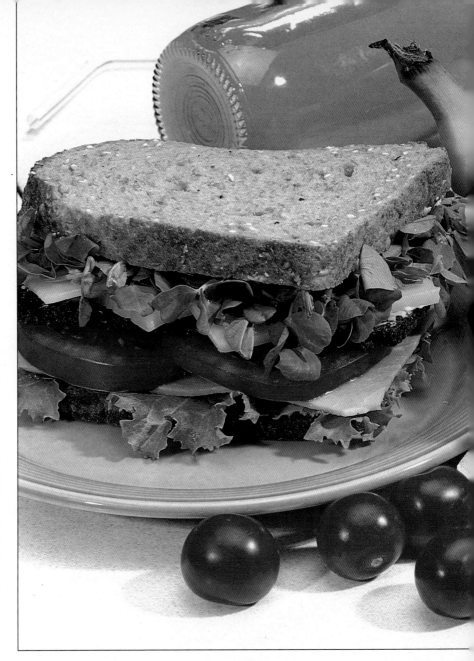

Health Club Sandwiches

● Canned tuna, salmon or sardines with lettuce, celery, green spring onions, sprouts, mixed salad, tomato, gherkin, reduced-fat mayonnaise, grated carrot, or cucumber.

● Peanut butter (try no-added-salt) with banana, honey, carrot and alfalfa, or cottage cheese and raisins.

● Corn with reduced-fat-and-salt ham and lettuce, or grated cheese, or chives and radish.

● Baked beans or bean mixes with lettuce and grated cheese or sliced onion and mushroom.

TASTY TOPPERS

Bread, muffins and crumpets topped with favourite foods are quick and easy and add extra carbohydrate and energy. For quick topping ideas try the following:

● Spaghetti, baked beans or corn kernels, no-added-salt.

● Low-fat cottage cheese with raisins and nuts.

● Mashed bananas and cinnamon.

● Low-fat cottage cheese and fruit chutney.

● Peanut butter and honey.

● Grilled pineapple and cheese.

● Mashed pumpkin or parsnip and cracked pepper.

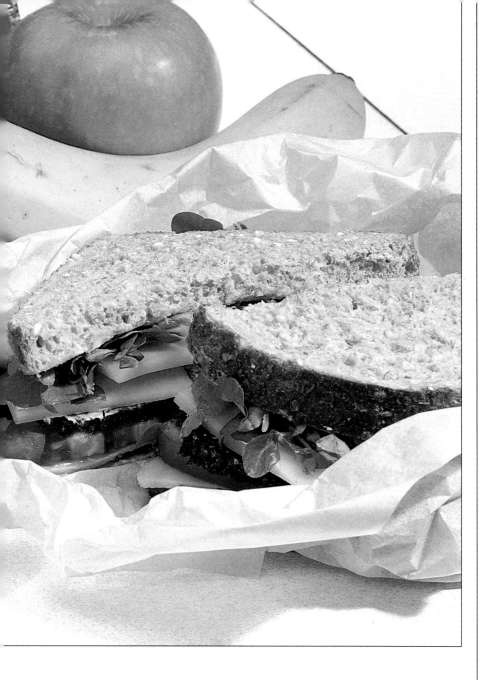

HEALTH CLUB SANDWICHES

Serves 4

- ☐ **1 tablespoon margarine**
- ☐ **4 slices wholegrain bread**
- ☐ **4 slices rye bread**
- ☐ **1 curly endive**
- ☐ **4 slices lean ham**
- ☐ **2 tomatoes, sliced**
- ☐ **4 slices reduced-fat cheddar cheese**
- ☐ **½ bunch watercress**
- ☐ **4 slices pumpernickel**

1　Spread margarine thinly on one side of each slice of wholegrain and rye bread. Top rye bread with endive, ham and tomatoes then slices of pumpernickel bread.

2　Place cheese and watercress on rye bread and top with wholegrain bread. Cut each sandwich in half and serve immediately.

450 Calories (1895 kilojoules) per serve

Carbohydrate	*56.0 g*	*Medium*
Protein	*27.0 g*	
Fat	*12.5 g*	*Medium*
Fibre	*8.5 g*	*High*

● Preparing lunch for school or work the night before will help avoid the morning rush.

● Lunch should include a variety of foods and supply about one-third of your daily nutrient needs.

● In summer, try salad boxes. Team a variety of salads with cold meat or chicken, cheese, canned tuna or salmon, or boiled eggs and fresh fruit.

● To keep summer lunches cool, pack frozen fruit pieces or fruit drinks in the container next to the salads and sandwiches.

● In winter, use a vacuum flask for soups, stews or casseroles.

● For those who have higher energy require-ments, add to lunches: dried fruit and nut mix, healthy biscuits, slices or muffins, low-fat yogurt, fruit juices and cheese sticks.

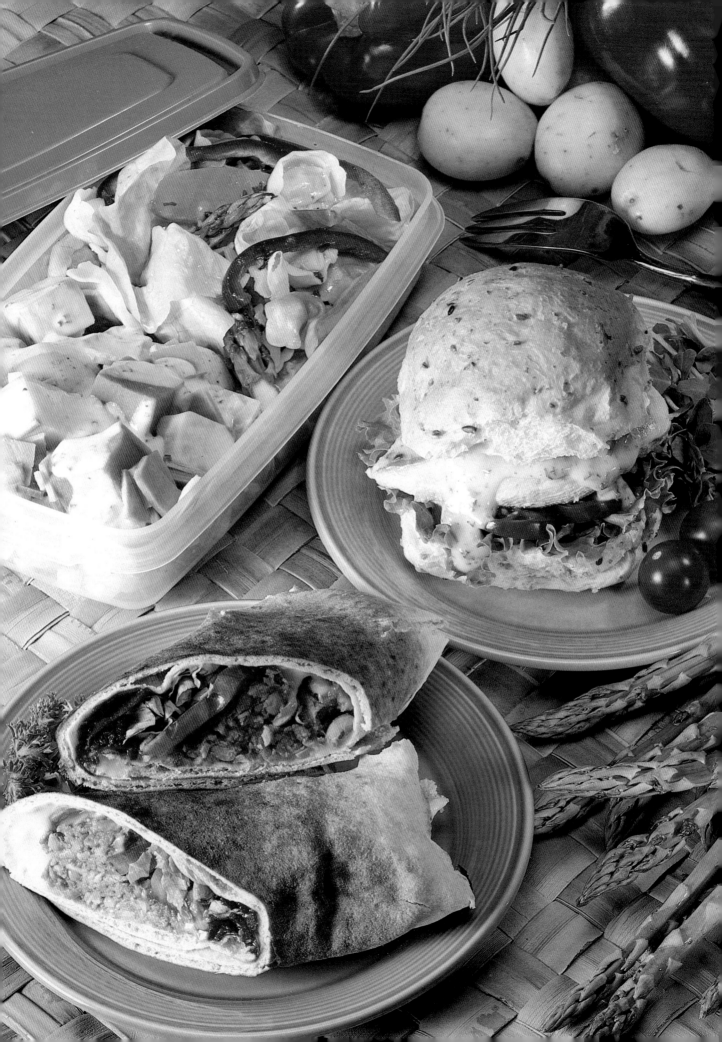

VEGETABLE AND SALAD ROLL-UPS

Serves 4

- ☐ **4 wholemeal pitta bread rounds or naan bread**
- ☐ **4 tablespoons reduced-fat mayonnaise**
- ☐ **8 lettuce leaves, shredded**
- ☐ **2 tomatoes, sliced**
- ☐ **1 beetroot, peeled and grated**

BEAN PATTIES
- ☐ **60 g (2 oz) wholemeal breadcrumbs, made from stale bread**
- ☐ **440 g (14 oz) canned haricot or cannelini beans, drained and roughly mashed**
- ☐ **1 carrot, grated**
- ☐ **1 courgette, grated**
- ☐ **2 tablespoons tomato puree**
- ☐ **¹/₂ teaspoon ground cumin**
- ☐ **1 egg white**

1   To make patties, place breadcrumbs, beans, carrot, courgette, tomato puree, cumin and egg white in a bowl and mix to combine. Shape mixture into 12 small patties and cook in a nonstick frying pan, for 3 minutes each side or until golden brown. Set aside to keep warm.
2   Spread bread rounds with mayonnaise. Top with lettuce, tomato, beetroot and patties. Roll up bread to form a cylinder and serve immediately.

205 Calories (855 kilojoules) per serve
Carbohydrate	*27.0 g*	*Medium*
Protein	*13.0 g*	
Fat	*4.0 g*	*Low*
Fibre	*13.4 g*	*High*

TORTELLINI SALAD

Serves 4

- ☐ **750 g (1¹/₂ lb) mixed-coloured meat-filled tortellini**
- ☐ **250 g (8 oz) asparagus, cut into 5 cm (2 in) pieces**
- ☐ **220 g (7 oz) mangetout, trimmed**
- ☐ **1 lettuce**
- ☐ **1 red pepper, sliced**
- ☐ **250 g (8 oz) yellow cherry tomatoes**
- ☐ **125 mL (4 fl oz) no-oil Italian dressing**

1   Cook tortellini in boiling water in a large saucepan, following packet directions. Drain, rinse under cold water and set aside to cool.
2   Boil, steam or microwave asparagus and mangetout separately until tender. Refresh under cold running water and set aside to cool.
3   Arrange lettuce, red pepper, tomatoes, tortellini, asparagus and mangetout in large serving bowl. Pour dressing over and serve immediately.
Do ahead: Cook the pasta and vegetables for this salad in advance and store in the refrigerator for up to 2 days. The salad then only takes minutes to assemble.

445 Calories (1860 kilojoules) per serve
Carbohydrate	*72.0 g*	*High*
Protein	*29.0 g*	
Fat	*3.0 g*	*Low*
Fibre	*9.0 g*	*High*

HERB AND CHICKEN BURGERS

Serves 4

- ☐ **4 chicken breast fillets, approximately 125 g (4 oz) each**
- ☐ **4 round, wholegrain bread rolls, halved and toasted**
- ☐ **12 cherry tomatoes, sliced**
- ☐ **1 curly endive lettuce**

HERB MAYONNAISE
- ☐ **4 tablespoons reduced-fat mayonnaise**
- ☐ **2 teaspoons snipped fresh chives**
- ☐ **2 teaspoons chopped fresh parsley**

1   To make mayonnaise, place mayonnaise, chives and parsley in a bowl and mix to combine.
2   Heat a large nonstick frying pan and cook chicken, for 4-5 minutes each side, or until golden and tender. Place a chicken breast on base of each roll. Top with tomato and lettuce. Spoon mayonnaise over and top with remaining roll halves.
Serving suggestion: Serve with coleslaw and fresh fruit.

510 Calories (2140 kilojoules) per serve
Carbohydrate	*55.0 g*	*Low*
Protein	*41.0 g*	
Fat	*13.0 g*	*Medium*
Fibre	*7.2 g*	*High*

TRI-POTATO SALAD

Serves 4

 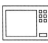

- ☐ **12 baby new potatoes**
- ☐ **500 g (1 lb) orange sweet potato, peeled and cubed**
- ☐ **500 g (1 lb) white potato, peeled and cubed**
- ☐ **1 small onion, chopped**
- ☐ **250 g (8 oz) lean ham, chopped**

MUSTARD HERB DRESSING
- ☐ **5 tablespoons reduced-fat mayonnaise**
- ☐ **3 tablespoons low-fat natural yogurt**
- ☐ **2 teaspoons wholegrain mustard**
- ☐ **2 tablespoons snipped fresh chives**

1   Boil, steam or microwave baby potatoes and sweet and white potatoes separately, until tender. Drain and set aside to keep warm.
2   Heat a nonstick frying pan and cook onion and ham for 3 minutes or until onion is soft.
3   Place potatoes in a large serving bowl and toss through onion mixture.
4   To make dressing, place mayonnaise, yogurt, mustard and chives in a bowl and mix to combine. Spoon over warm salad and serve.
Serving suggestion: A salad of oranges and onions tossed in Fast French Dressing (see page 28) is a good accompaniment for this salad.

410 Calories (1730 kilojoules) per serve
Carbohydrate	*58.0 g*	*Medium*
Protein	*25.0 g*	
Fat	*9.0 g*	*Low*
Fibre	*10.8 g*	*High*

*Tortellini Salad, Tri-Potato Salad,
Herb and Chicken Burgers, Vegetable and
Salad Roll-Ups*

Pyramid power

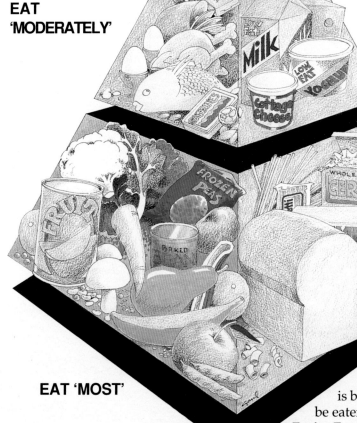

EAT 'IN SMALL AMOUNTS' FOODS

EAT 'IN SMALL AMOUNTS'

Fats and oils: Butter, margarine, cooking oil and salad dressings. To reduce cholesterol, choose mono-unsaturated (olive, peanut or soya oil) or polyunsaturated fats (margarine – including reduced fat varieties – sunflower and safflower oils).

Sugar and sugar-based foods: Confectionery, soft drinks, desserts, honey and jams. Sugar-based foods are often used by active people to top up energy stores, but, unfortunately, many of these foods contain excess fat. A small amount of sugar does no harm.

EAT 'MODERATELY' FOODS

EAT 'MODERATELY'

These foods provide much of the protein in your diet and are essential for growth and repair of tissues.

Meat, poultry, seafood, eggs: An excellent source of good quality protein. Reduce fat by choosing lean meats and removing skin from poultry. Avoid cooking in fat.

Nuts: The protein contained in these is of a poorer quality to the proteins above. Improve quality by eating nuts in combination with grains or seeds.

Dairy foods: Include, milk, cheese and yogurt. To decrease fat intake use reduced- or low-fat types.

EAT 'MOST' FOODS

EAT 'MOST'

These foods are rich in complex carbohydrate and fibre, low in fat and make the ideal fuel for peak performance.

Breads and cereals: Rich in carbohydrate, fibre and B vitamins. Eat as meals or snacks. Wholegrain is best. Remember breakfast cereal does not just have to be eaten at breakfast.

Fruits: Eat a variety to provide a range of essential vitamins. Fruit is a convenient snack.

Vegetables: With the exception of potatoes and legumes (dried peas, beans, lentils), vegetables do not contain as much carbohydrate as breads, cereals or fruit. They are an excellent source of vitamins, minerals and fibre. Eat a variety of different coloured vegetables to provide a range of essential nutrients.

*The Healthy Diet Pyramid – reproduced
courtesy of the Australian Nutrition Foundation*

Energise for exercise

Just as a car burns fuel, people burn up food in their body to give them energy.

The fuel, or energy value in food and the amount of energy we use, is measured in calories (kilojoules). It is important to realise that these requirements can vary quite substantially from person to person. It is possible to calculate the approximate amount of energy burnt during exercise. This table is a guide to the approximate amount of energy used during various sporting activities.

● Age, sex, body size/ weight and physical activity affect the energy we use.
● A stable bodyweight is perhaps the best guide as to how well your energy requirements are being met.
● Consuming too much energy causes increased weight.
● Too little energy intake causes weight loss.

ACTIVITIES	BODYWEIGHT				
Per Minute	50 kg (110 lb) cals (kJ)	56 kg (123 lb) cals (kJ)	59 kg (130 lb) cals (kJ)	71 kg (157 lb) cals (kJ)	80 kg (176 lb) cals (kJ)
Aerobics	5.2 (21.8)	5.8 (24.3)	6.1 (25.5)	7.3 (30.6)	8.2 (34.3)
Basketball	6.9 (28.9)	7.7 (32.2)	8.1 (33.9)	9.8 (41.0)	11.0 (46.0)
Circuit Training					
Universal	5.8 (24.3)	6.5 (27.2)	6.9 (28.9)	8.3 (34.7)	9.3 (38.9)
Nautilus	4.6 (19.3)	5.2 (21.8)	5.5 (23.0)	6.6 (27.6)	7.4 (31.0)
Free Weights	4.3 (18.0)	4.8 (20.1)	5.0 (20.9)	6.1 (25.5)	6.8 (28.5)
Cricket	4.5 (18.8)	5.0 (20.9)	5.3 (22.2)	6.4 (26.8)	7.2 (30.1)
Cycling					
Leisure	3.2 (13.4)	3.6 (15.1)	3.8 (15.9)	4.5 (18.8)	5.1 (21.3)
Racing	8.5 (35.6)	9.5 (39.8)	10 (41.9)	12.0 (50.2)	13.5 (56.5)
Football	6.6 (27.6)	7.4 (31.0)	7.8 (32.7)	9.4 (39.3)	10.6 (44.4)
Golf	4.3 (18.0)	4.8 (20.1)	5.0 (21.0)	6.0 (25.1)	6.8 (28.5)
Gymnastics	3.3 (13.8)	3.7 (15.5)	3.9 (10.3)	4.7 (19.7)	5.3 (22.2)
Cross Country Running	8.2 (34.3)	9.1 (38.1)	9.6 (40.2)	11.6 (48.6)	13.0 (54.4)
Running					
7 min/km (11 min/mile)	6.8 (28.5)	7.6 (31.8)	8.0 (33.5)	9.6 (40.2)	10.9 (45.6)
Cross Country Skiing	6.0 (25.1)	6.7 (28.0)	7.0 (29.3)	8.4 (35.2)	9.5 (39.8)
Squash	10.6 (44.4)	11.9 (49.8)	12.5 (52.3)	15.1 (63.2)	17.0 (71.2)
Swimming					
Freestyle (fast)	7.8 (32.7)	8.7 (36.4)	9.2 (38.5)	11.1 (46.5)	12.5 (52.3)
Backstroke	8.5 (35.6)	9.5 (39.8)	10.0 (41.9)	12.0 (50.2)	13.5 (56.5)
Breaststroke	8.1 (33.9)	9.1 (39.1)	9.6 (40.2)	11.5 (48.1)	13.0 (54.4)
Tennis	5.5 (23.0)	6.1 (25.5)	6.4 (26.8)	7.7 (32.2)	8.7 (36.4)
Walking (medium pace)	4.0 (16.7)	4.5 (18.8)	4.7 (19.7)	5.7 (23.9)	6.4 (26.8)

Adapted from McArdle W.P., Katch I.F. and Katch V.C. Exercise Physiology Energy, Nutrition and Human Performance, Lea and Febiger, Philadelphia, 1986

Mighty mains

FISH CAKES WITH CHILLI SAUCE

Serves 4

- [ ] **500 g (1 lb) boneless white fish fillets**
- [ ] **1 clove garlic, crushed**
- [ ] **60 g (2 oz) wholemeal breadcrumbs, made from stale bread**
- [ ] **1 egg white**
- [ ] **2 spring onions, finely chopped**
- [ ] **1 tablespoon lemon juice**
- [ ] **2 tablespoons low-fat natural yogurt**

CHILLI SAUCE
- [ ] **1 teaspoon olive oil**
- [ ] **3 spring onions, chopped**
- [ ] **1/2 red pepper, finely chopped**
- [ ] **1 red chilli, seeded and finely chopped**
- [ ] **440 g (14 oz) canned peeled tomatoes, no-added-salt, drained and chopped**
- [ ] **250 mL (8 fl oz) creamed tomatoes, no-added-salt**

1   Place fish in a food processor and process until smooth. Add garlic, breadcrumbs, egg white, spring onions, lemon juice and yogurt and mix to combine.
2   Wet hands and shape mixture into 8 patties. Heat a nonstick frying pan and cook patties over a medium heat for 2-3 minutes each side. Remove from pan and set aside to keep warm.
3   To make sauce, heat oil in a saucepan and cook spring onions, red pepper and chilli for 3-4 minutes. Add tomatoes and creamed tomatoes, bring to the boil, then reduce heat and simmer uncovered, for 5 minutes or until sauce thickens slightly.
Serving suggestion: Top patties with Chilli Sauce and accompany with brown rice and a crisp green salad. These fish cakes

can also be served in a wholemeal roll. Split the roll and toast cut sides. On bottom half of roll place a lettuce leaf, a fish cake and a spoonful of Chilli Sauce, then top of roll.
Do ahead: The uncooked fish cakes can be stored in the refrigerator for up to a day, or frozen for up to two months.

205 Calories (860 kilojoules) per serve
Carbohydrate	*12.0 g*	*Low*
Protein	*28.0 g*	
Fat	*5.0 g*	*Low*
Fibre	*2.4 g*	*Medium*

VEGETARIAN PAN PIZZA

Serves 4

- [ ] **15 g (1/2 oz) fresh yeast**
- [ ] **1/2 teaspoon sugar**
- [ ] **125 mL (4 fl oz) lukewarm water**
- [ ] **220 g (7 oz) wholemeal flour, sifted and husks returned**
- [ ] **1 teaspoon olive oil**

AUBERGINE AND HERB TOPPING
- [ ] **1 small aubergine, finely sliced**
- [ ] **2 teaspoons olive oil**
- [ ] **4 tablespoons tomato sauce, no-added-salt**
- [ ] **1 teaspoon chopped fresh oregano**
- [ ] **1 teaspoon chopped fresh basil**
- [ ] **1 onion, finely sliced**
- [ ] **1 red pepper, finely sliced**
- [ ] **6 button mushrooms, finely sliced**
- [ ] **200 g (6 1/2 oz) canned pineapple pieces, drained**
- [ ] **4 black olives, pitted and sliced**
- [ ] **60 g (2 oz) grated medium-fat mozzarella cheese**

1   Place yeast and sugar in a bowl and mix to combine. Stir in water, cover and stand in a warm place until mixture bubbles. Place flour in a separate bowl, stir in yeast mixture and oil and mix to a soft dough.
2   Turn dough onto a lightly floured

surface and knead for 5 minutes, or until dough is smooth and elastic. Place dough in a lightly oiled bowl, cover and set aside in a warm place for 30 minutes, or until dough has doubled in size.
3   Remove dough from bowl and knead on a lightly floured surface. Roll out dough to a 25 cm (10 in) circle and place in a nonstick 25 cm (10 in) frying pan.
4   To make topping, brush aubergine slices with oil and cook under a preheated grill until brown each side. Spread dough with tomato sauce then sprinkle with oregano and basil. Top with aubergine, onion, red pepper, mushrooms, pineapple, olives and cheese.
5   Cover pan and cook over a low heat for 35 minutes, or until pizza crust is cooked. Place pizza under a preheated grill for 3 minutes, or until cheese melts and is golden.
Variation: This is a vegetarian pizza, but you can vary the topping according to what you have and what your favourite foods are. If you want to add some meat or fish you might like to use some chopped lean ham, or canned tuna in water, drained, in place of the aubergine.
Serving suggestion: Cut pizza into wedges and serve with coleslaw or a green salad, and crusty bread rolls.

310 Calories (1300 kilojoules) per serve
Carbohydrate	*46.0 g*	*High*
Protein	*13.0 g*	
Fat	*8.0 g*	*Medium*
Fibre	*7.3 g*	*High*

Minestrone Soup (page 24), Vegetarian Pan Pizza, Fish Cakes with Chilli Sauce

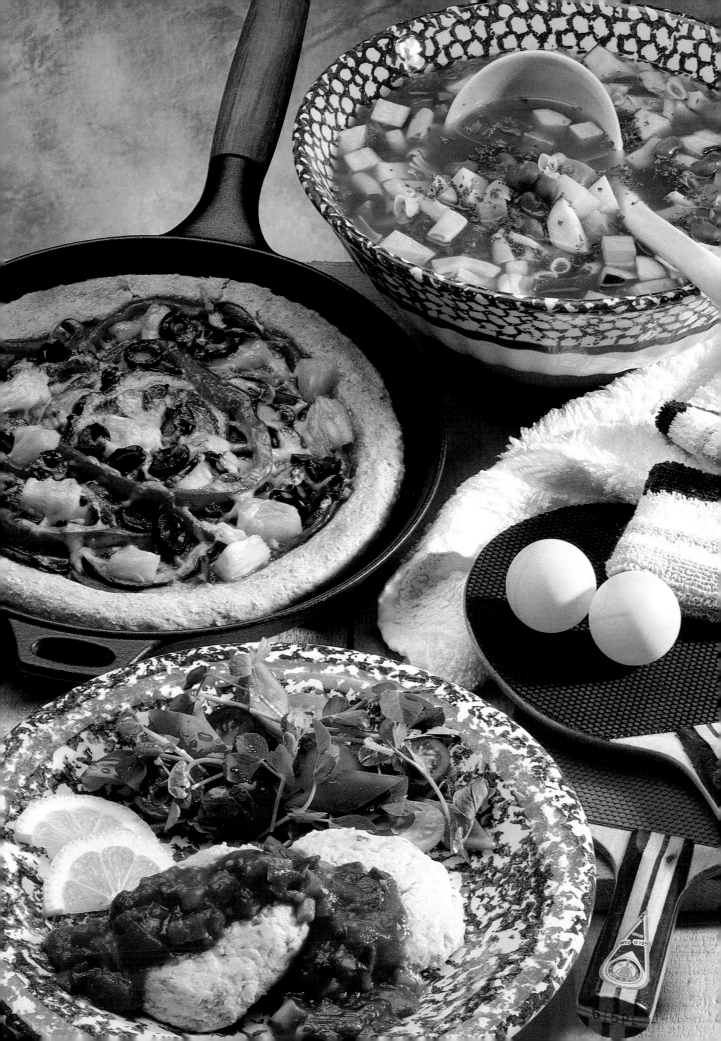

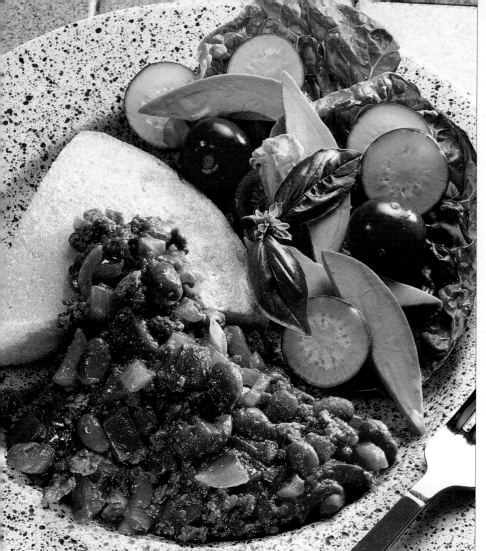

CHILLI CON CARNE WITH CORN BREAD

Serves 4
Oven temperature 180°C, 350°F, Gas 4

- ☐ 2 onions, chopped
- ☐ 2 cloves garlic, crushed
- ☐ ¹/₂ red pepper, finely chopped
- ☐ 440 g (14 oz) canned peeled tomatoes, no-added-salt, drained, chopped and 1 tablespoon juice reserved
- ☐ 500 g (1 lb) lean minced beef
- ☐ ¹/₂ teaspoon chilli powder
- ☐ 1 teaspoon ground cumin
- ☐ 1 teaspoon ground coriander
- ☐ 2 tablespoons tomato puree, no-added-salt
- ☐ 315 g (10 oz) canned red kidney beans, drained and rinsed
- ☐ 125 mL (4 fl oz) beef stock

CORN BREAD
- ☐ 185 g (6 oz) polenta (corn meal)
- ☐ 90 g (3 oz) self-raising flour, sifted
- ☐ ¹/₂ teaspoon sugar
- ☐ 1 tablespoon polyunsaturated margarine, melted
- ☐ 250 mL (8 fl oz) skimmed milk
- ☐ 1 egg

1   Heat a nonstick frying pan and cook onions, garlic, red pepper and reserved juice from tomatoes over a medium heat for 4-5 minutes. Stir in mince and cook for 10 minutes longer. Add tomatoes, chilli powder, cumin, coriander, tomato puree, red kidney beans and stock. Bring to the boil, then reduce heat and simmer for 25 minutes.
2   To make Corn Bread, combine polenta, flour and sugar in a bowl. Whisk together margarine, milk and egg and stir into polenta mixture. Mix to combine ingredients.
3   Spread mixture into a greased 20 cm (8 in) round cake pan and bake for 15-20 minutes, or until bread is golden. Serve warm with Chilli Con Carne.

605 Calories (2545 kilojoules) per serve

Carbohydrate	*66.0 g*	*Low*
Protein	*50.0 g*	
Fat	*15.0 g*	*Medium*
Fibre	*12.1 g*	*High*

MINESTRONE SOUP

Serves 4

- ☐ 1 onion, chopped
- ☐ 3 cloves garlic, crushed
- ☐ 2 x 440 g (14 oz) canned peeled tomatoes, no-added-salt, undrained and chopped
- ☐ 1 large potato, peeled and cut into small cubes
- ☐ 2 courgette, cut into small cubes
- ☐ 2 carrots, peeled, cut into small cubes
- ☐ freshly ground black pepper
- ☐ 1 teaspoon dried oregano
- ☐ 2 teaspoons dried basil
- ☐ 1 litre (1³/₄ pt) vegetable stock
- ☐ 400 g (14 oz) canned red kidney beans, drained and rinsed
- ☐ 155 g (5 oz) macaroni, cooked and drained
- ☐ 1 tablespoon chopped fresh parsley
- ☐ 2 tablespoons grated fresh Parmesan cheese

1   Place onion, garlic and 2 tablespoons of juice from tomatoes in a saucepan and cook over a medium heat for 2-3 minutes, or until onion is soft. Add potato, courgette, carrots, black pepper to taste, oregano, and basil and cook, uncovered, for 5 minutes, stirring frequently.
2   Stir in tomatoes and stock, bring to the boil, then reduce heat and simmer, uncovered, for 20 minutes.
3   Add beans, macaroni and parsley and cook over a low heat for 5 minutes longer, or until heated through.
Serving suggestion: Ladle soup into serving bowls and sprinkle with Parmesan cheese. Serve with a crisp green salad and crusty wholemeal bread rolls.

205 Calories (855 kilojoules) per serve

Carbohydrate	*28.0 g*	*Medium*
Protein	*16.0 g*	
Fat	*2.0 g*	*Low*
Fibre	*2.9 g*	*High*

AUBERGINE LASAGNE

Serves 4
Oven temperature 180°C, 350°F, Gas 4

- [ ] 1 tablespoon olive oil
- [ ] ½ teaspoon freshly ground black pepper
- [ ] 3 tablespoons lemon juice
- [ ] 1 large aubergine, about 500 g (1 lb), halved lengthways and cut into ½ cm (¼ in) thick slices
- [ ] 30 g (1 oz) wholemeal breadcrumbs, made from stale bread
- [ ] 3 tablespoons grated Parmesan cheese
- [ ] 1 large onion, chopped
- [ ] 2 cloves garlic, crushed
- [ ] 440 g (14 oz) canned peeled tomatoes, no-added-salt, drained, chopped and 1 tablespoon juice reserved
- [ ] 185 mL (6 fl oz) creamed tomatoes, no-added-salt
- [ ] 2 tablespoons white wine
- [ ] 1 teaspoon dried oregano
- [ ] 1 teaspoon dried basil
- [ ] pinch cayenne pepper
- [ ] 6 wholemeal ready-to-use lasagne sheets
- [ ] 185 g (6 oz) ricotta cheese
- [ ] 3 tablespoons grated medium-fat mozzarella cheese

1   Combine olive oil, black pepper and lemon juice and brush aubergine slices. Cook under preheated grill for 3-4 minutes each side or until golden. Combine breadcrumbs and Parmesan cheese and set aside.

2   Heat a nonstick frying pan and cook onion, garlic and reserved tomato juice over a medium heat for 2-3 minutes. Add peeled and creamed tomatoes, wine, oregano, basil and cayenne pepper and cook for 5 minutes longer.

3   Spread one-third of the tomato mixture over base of a 15 x 25 cm (6 x 10 in) ovenproof dish. Top with 3 lasagne sheets, half of the breadcrumb mixture and cover with a layer of aubergine. Top with half the ricotta cheese. Repeat layers, ending with a layer of tomato mixture. Top with mozzarella cheese and bake for 45 minutes.

285 Calories (1200 kilojoules) per serve

Carbohydrate	*27.0 g*	*Low*
Protein	*16.0 g*	
Fat	*13.0 g*	*High*
Fibre	*5.5 g*	*Medium*

Below: Aubergine Lasagne
Left: Chilli Con Carne with Corn Bread

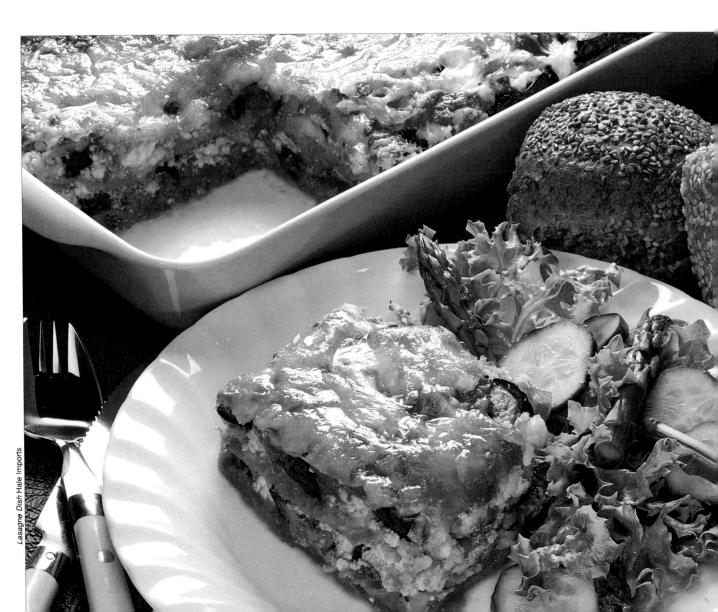

Lasagne Dish Hale Imports

GOLDEN SOUP

Serves 4

- ☐ 1 onion, chopped
- ☐ 1 clove garlic, crushed
- ☐ 1 litre (1³/₄ pt) chicken or vegetable stock
- ☐ 2 medium potatoes, peeled and sliced
- ☐ 750 g (1¹/₂ lb) pumpkin or carrot, peeled and sliced
- ☐ ¹/₂ teaspoon dried marjoram
- ☐ ¹/₂ teaspoon ground nutmeg
- ☐ freshly ground black pepper
- ☐ 3 tablespoons buttermilk or skimmed milk

1 Cook onion, garlic and 2 tablespoons stock in a large saucepan for 2-3 minutes, or until onion is soft. Add remaining stock, potatoes, pumpkin, marjoram, nutmeg, and black pepper to taste. Cook over a medium heat, stirring occasionally, for 25 minutes, or until pumpkin and potato are tender. Stir in buttermilk or skimmed milk, then remove from heat and set aside to cool slightly.

2 Transfer soup mixture in batches to a food processor or blender and process until smooth.

3 Return soup to a clean saucepan and heat gently, do not allow to boil or soup will curdle.

Serving suggestion: Pour soup into large mugs, sprinkle with snipped fresh chives and serve with wholegrain bread rolls.

Do ahead: The soup can be stored in the refrigerator for up to 3 days and reheated as required either in a saucepan or in the microwave. If reheating in the microwave you can reheat the soup in the serving mugs. One serving will take 2-3 minutes to reheat on HIGH (100%) – this time will depend on the serving size.

125 Calories (515 kilojoules) per serve

Carbohydrate	*21.5 g*	*High*
Protein	*6.5 g*	
Fat	*neg*	*Low*
Fibre	*2.4 g*	*Medium*

PORK FILLETS WITH RED WINE SAUCE

Serves 4

- ☐ 2 small pork fillets, each about 250 g (8 oz), trimmed of all visible fat
- ☐ 1 tablespoon honey, warmed
- ☐ 1 tablespoon Worcestershire sauce
- ☐ 1 tablespoon red wine

RED WINE SAUCE
- ☐ 1 small onion, chopped
- ☐ ¹/₂ stalk celery, chopped
- ☐ 250 mL (8 fl oz) chicken stock
- ☐ 1 teaspoon sweet fruit chutney
- ☐ 3 tablespoons red wine
- ☐ 2 teaspoons polyunsaturated margarine
- ☐ 2 teaspoons plain flour
- ☐ 220 g (7 oz) button mushrooms, sliced

1 Place fillets in a shallow dish. Combine honey, Worcestershire sauce and wine, pour over fillets and marinate for 15-20 minutes, turning occasionally. Cook on a hot barbecue or grill until tender, brushing several times with marinade during cooking.

2 To make sauce, place onion, celery, stock, chutney and red wine in a saucepan and cook over a low heat for 5 minutes, or until liquid is reduced by half. Strain and set aside.

3 Melt margarine in a clean saucepan, stir in flour and cook over a medium heat for 1 minute. Remove pan from heat and gradually whisk in red wine mixture. Add mushrooms and cook, stirring constantly, until sauce boils and thickens.

Serving suggestion: Slice pork fillets and spoon sauce over. Serve with a green salad and boiled new potatoes.

275 Calories (1150 kilojoules) per serve

Carbohydrate	*10.0 g*	*Low*
Protein	*29.0 g*	
Fat	*12.0 g*	*High*
Fibre	*1.5 g*	*Low*

QUICK AND EASY QUICHE

Serves 4
Oven temperature 180°C, 350°F, Gas 4

- ☐ 15 g (¹/₂ oz) polyunsaturated margarine, melted
- ☐ 8 slices wholegrain bread, crusts removed

FILLING
- ☐ 155 g (5 oz) broccoli, cut into florets
- ☐ ¹/₂ red pepper, chopped
- ☐ 125 g (4 oz) canned sweet corn kernels, drained
- ☐ 90 g (3 oz) button mushrooms, sliced
- ☐ 4 eggs, lightly beaten
- ☐ 185 mL (6 fl oz) skimmed milk
- ☐ 60 g (2 oz) grated reduced-fat cheddar cheese
- ☐ freshly ground black pepper

1 Brush a 23 cm (9 in) flan dish with margarine. Line dish with bread, trimming slices to fit base and sides.

2 To make filling, arrange broccoli, red pepper, sweet corn and mushrooms over bread. Combine eggs and milk and pour over vegetables. Sprinkle with cheese, and black pepper to taste. Bake for 30-35 minutes, or until filling is firm.

Serving suggestion: Can be served hot, warm or cold with vegetables or salad.

330 Calories (1385 kilojoules) per serve

Carbohydrate	*30.0 g*	*Low*
Protein	*21.0 g*	
Fat	*14.0 g*	*High*
Fibre	*7.0 g*	*High*

POLENTA

Polenta is a maize flour much used in Italy for both savoury and sweet dishes. It is available in most supermarkets, Italian food stores and health-food shops. The grainy texture of cooked polenta may surprise you at first, but that's how it's meant to be.

Golden Butternut Soup, Pork Fillets with Red Wine Sauce, Quick and Easy Quiche

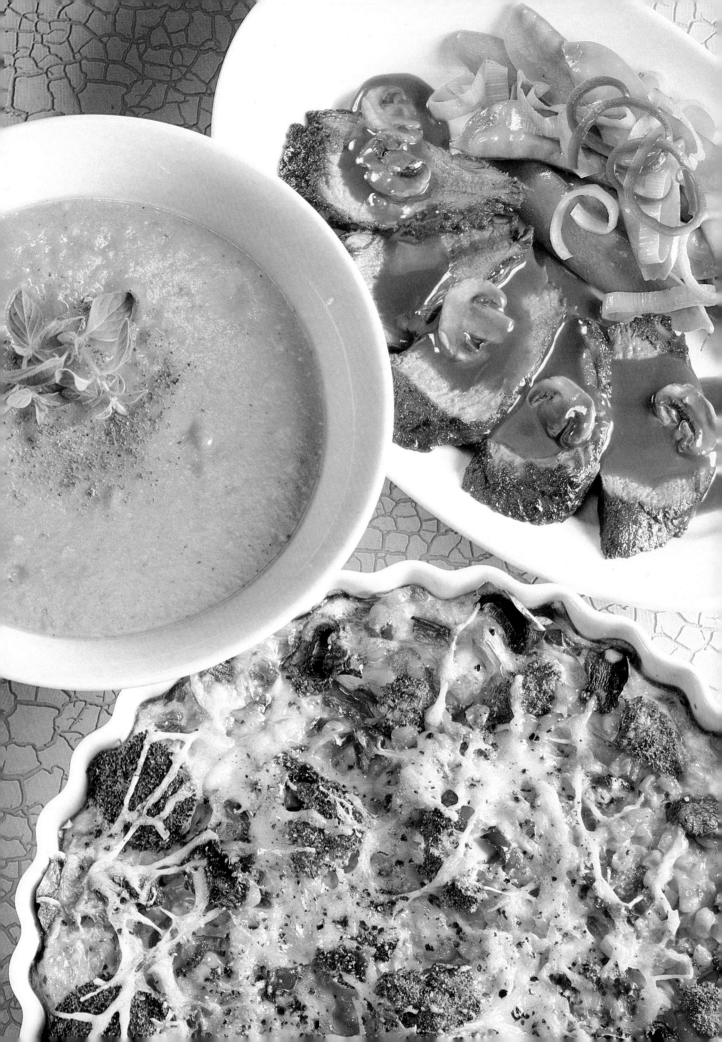

DRESS UP A SALAD

An interesting dressing is all that is needed to turn a salad into something special.

● Make a larger quantity of dressing than you need so that you always have some on hand. Store in a bottle or screwtop jar in the refrigerator.

● Some dressings are also good served as a dip to go with raw or lightly cooked vegetable sticks, while others are delicious tossed through hot pasta.

● Many salads do not require a recipe if you have a few basic ingredients and an interesting dressing. Try some of the following ideas then use your imagination to make your own salads.

● **Potato salad:** Cook extra potatoes when cooking the evening meal, allow to cool and store in the refrigerator. Make the salad by cutting the potatoes in pieces then tossing in a dressing.

● **Hot potato salad** is a good alternative when you do not have any cold potatoes, boil or microwave potatoes, cut into pieces and toss in a dressing. If using small new potatoes, they only need to be scrubbed then cooked and can be left whole or halved.

● **Quick lettuce salads** are easy to make if you keep 2 to 3 different types of lettuce and a few fresh herbs, on hand. To make the salad, take a few leaves from each lettuce, wash and dry, tear into pieces and place in a salad bowl, add chopped fresh herbs and toss with a dressing.

● **Coleslaw** is easily made by shredding cabbage and combining it with grated carrot, diced red or green pepper, diced celery and chopped fresh herbs, then tossing through a dressing.

Note: A serve for all dressings in this book is one tablespoon

ORIENTAL DRESSING

Makes 250 mL (8 fl oz)

- ☐ **2 tablespoons polyunsaturated vegetable oil**
- ☐ **¹/₂ teaspoon sesame oil**
- ☐ **1 tablespoon sweet sherry**
- ☐ **1 tablespoon soy sauce**
- ☐ **2 teaspoons grated fresh ginger**
- ☐ **1 tablespoon sesame seeds**
- ☐ **1 small chilli, finely chopped**

Place vegetable oil, sesame oil, sherry, soy sauce, ginger, sesame seeds and chilli in a screwtop jar. Shake well to combine.

Serving suggestion: Use as a dressing on a salad made from Chinese noodles, pasta or lettuce. Also delicious tossed through hot noodles for a quick flavour booster.

35 Calories (155 kilojoules) per serve
Carbohydrate	*neg*	*Low*
Protein	*neg*	
Fat	*4.0 g*	*High*
Fibre	*neg*	*Low*

FAST FRENCH DRESSING

Makes 250 mL (8 fl oz)

- ☐ **2 tablespoons olive oil**
- ☐ **4 tablespoons lemon or lime juice**
- ☐ **4 tablespoons white wine vinegar**
- ☐ **¹/₄ teaspoon dry mustard powder**
- ☐ **¹/₂ teaspoon sugar**
- ☐ **1 tablespoon finely chopped fresh parsley**
- ☐ **1 tablespoon snipped fresh chives**
- ☐ **1 tablespoon chopped fresh tarragon**

Place olive oil, lemon or lime juice, vinegar, mustard powder, sugar, parsley, chives and tarragon in a screwtop jar. Shake well to combine.

Serving suggestion: Use as a dressing on coleslaw, lettuce or hot potato salad.

25 Calories(115 kilojoules) per serve
Carbohydrate	*neg*	*Low*
Protein	*neg*	
Fat	*3.0 g*	*High*
Fibre	*neg*	*Low*

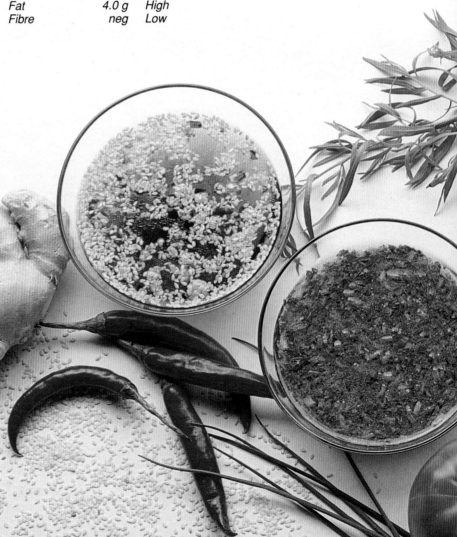

ISLAND HOPPING DRESSING

Makes 250 mL (8 fl oz)

- ☐ **4 tablespoons low-fat natural yogurt**
- ☐ **2 tablespoons skimmed milk**
- ☐ **1 tablespoon tomato puree, no-added-salt**
- ☐ **1 tablespoon red wine vinegar**
- ☐ **3 drops Tabasco sauce**

Place yogurt, milk, tomato puree, vinegar and Tabasco sauce in a screwtop jar. Shake well to combine.

Serving suggestion: Use as a dressing on coleslaw, potato or pasta salad. Also delicious served as a dip with raw or lightly cooked vegetable sticks.

10 Calories (50 kilojoules) per serve

Carbohydrate	1.5 g	Low
Protein	1.0 g	
Fat	neg	Low
Fibre	none	Low

PESTO DRESSING

Makes 250 mL (8 fl oz)

- ☐ **2 tablespoons vegetable oil**
- ☐ **4 tablespoons white vinegar**
- ☐ **60 g (2 oz) fresh basil leaves**
- ☐ **1 tablespoon pine nuts, toasted**
- ☐ **2 cloves garlic, peeled**
- ☐ **2 tablespoons grated fresh Parmesan cheese**

Place oil, vinegar, basil leaves, pine nuts, garlic and Parmesan cheese in a food processor or blender and process until smooth.

Serving suggestion: Use as a dressing on a mixed pasta salad. Also good as a dip for raw or lightly steamed vegetables and wonderful tossed through hot pasta.

45 Calories (185 kilojoules) per serve

Carbohydrate	neg	Low
Protein	1.0 g	
Fat	4.5 g	High
Fibre	neg	Low

TANGY CUCUMBER DRESSING

Makes 375 mL (12 fl oz)

- ☐ **200 g (6^1/$_2$ oz) low-fat natural yogurt**
- ☐ **1 small cucumber, seeded and finely chopped**
- ☐ **1 tablespoon wholegrain mustard**

Place yogurt, cucumber and mustard in a bowl and mix to combine.

Serving suggestion: Use as a dressing for potato salad, or as a dip for raw or lightly cooked vegetable sticks.

6 Calories (25 kilojoules) per serve

Carbohydrate	neg	Low
Protein	neg	
Fat	neg	Low
Fibre	neg	Low

From left: Oriental Dressing, Fast French Dressing, Island Hopping Dressing, Pesto Dressing, Tangy Cucumber Dressing

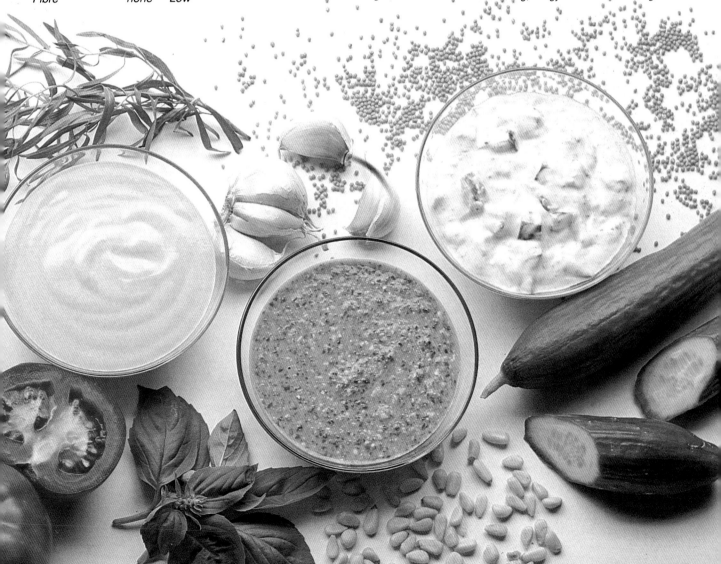

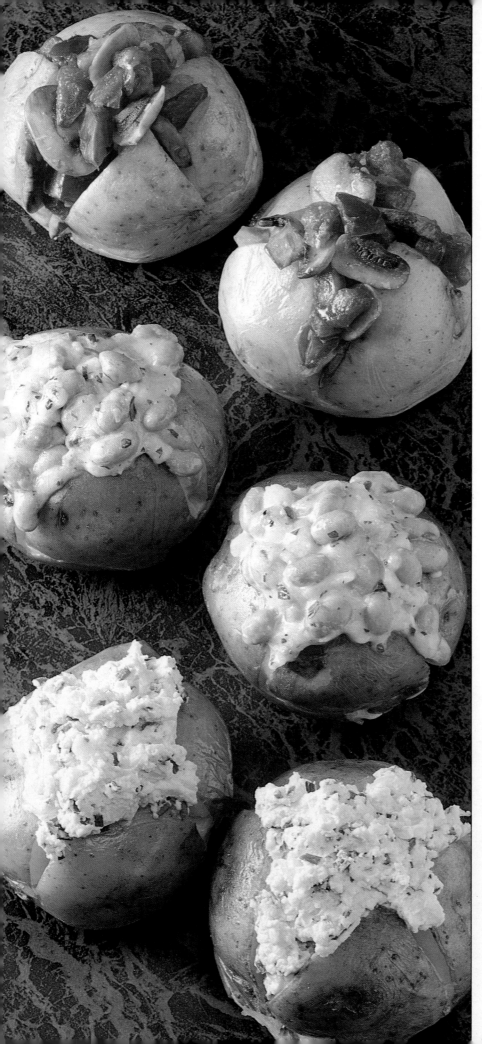

CHEESY TOPPED POTATOES

Serves 4

- ☐ **8 potatoes, scrubbed**

CHEESE AND CHIVE TOPPING
- ☐ **185 g (6 oz) reduced-fat ricotta cheese**
- ☐ **4 tablespoons grated reduced-fat cheddar cheese**
- ☐ **2 tablespoons snipped fresh chives**
- ☐ **freshly ground black pepper**

1   Boil, steam or microwave potatoes until tender.
2   To make topping, combine ricotta and cheddar cheeses, chives, and black pepper to taste in a bowl.
3   Cut a cross in the top of each potato and press to open out. Divide topping between potatoes and place under a preheated grill for 4-5 minutes, or until cheese melts and filling is warm.

190 Calories (790 kilojoules) per serve
Carbohydrate	*22.0 g*	*Low*
Protein	*11.0 g*	
Fat	*6.0 g*	*Medium*
Fibre	*4.5 g*	*Medium*

MUSHROOM TOPPED POTATOES

Serves 4

- ☐ **8 potatoes, scrubbed**

TOMATO AND MUSHROOM TOPPING
- ☐ **2 teaspoons polyunsaturated margarine**
- ☐ **1 small onion, chopped**
- ☐ **250 g (8 oz) button mushrooms, sliced**
- ☐ **1 large tomato, chopped**
- ☐ **1 tablespoon chopped fresh basil**
- ☐ **freshly ground black pepper**

Mushroom Topped Potatoes, Cheesy Bean Potatoes, Cheesy Topped Potatoes

1 Boil, steam or microwave potatoes until tender.

2 To make topping, melt margarine in a small saucepan and cook onion for 3-4 minutes or until soft. Add mushrooms and tomato and cook for 4-5 minutes longer. Stir basil through and season to taste with black pepper.

3 Cut a cross in the top of each potato and press to open out. Divide topping between cut potatoes and serve.

140 Calories (580 kilojoules) per serve

Carbohydrate	23.0 g	High
Protein	6.0 g	
Fat	6.0 g	Low
Fibre	7.0 g	High

CHEESY BEAN POTATOES

Serves 4

☐ **8 potatoes, scrubbed**

BEAN TOPPING
☐ **250 mL (8 fl oz) skimmed milk**
☐ **2 tablespoons cornflour**
☐ **375 g (12 oz) soya beans, drained, cooked**
☐ **60 g (2 oz) grated reduced-fat cheddar cheese**
☐ **2 tablespoons grated fresh Parmesan cheese**
☐ **¼ teaspoon ground nutmeg**
☐ **1 tablespoon chopped fresh parsley**
☐ **black pepper**

1 Boil, steam or microwave potatoes until tender.

2 To make topping, place 185 mL (6 fl oz) milk in a small saucepan and heat gently for 3-4 minutes without boiling. Combine cornflour with remaining milk and add to saucepan. Stir constantly until sauce thickens. Stir in soya beans, cheddar cheese, Parmesan cheese, and nutmeg and cook for 2-3 minutes longer, or until heated through. Stir in parsley and season to taste with black pepper.

3 Cut a cross in the top of each potato and press to open out. Divide topping between potatoes and serve immediately.

235 Calories (995 kilojoules) per serve

Carbohydrate	29.0 g	Medium
Protein	16.0 g	
Fat	6.0 g	Medium
Fibre	10.0 g	High

HOT CHICKEN AND POTATO CURRY

Serves 4

☐ **10 new potatoes, peeled and halved**
☐ **2 onions, cut into eighths**
☐ **1 clove garlic, crushed**
☐ **½ teaspoon curry paste (Vindaloo)**
☐ **440 g (14 oz) canned peeled tomatoes, no-added-salt, undrained and mashed**
☐ **250 mL (8 oz) chicken stock**
☐ **2 tablespoons dry white wine**
☐ **2 tablespoons mango chutney**
☐ **3 teaspoons curry powder**
☐ **2 teaspoons ground cumin**
☐ **4 tablespoons tomato puree, no-added-salt**
☐ **2 chicken breast fillets, cut into 2.5 cm (1 in) cubes**
☐ **1 tablespoon finely chopped fresh coriander**

1 Boil, steam or microwave potatoes until just tender. Set aside to cool.

2 Place onions, garlic, curry paste and 1 tablespoon of juice from tomatoes in a saucepan and cook for 2-3 minutes, or until onion is soft.

3 Combine tomatoes, stock, wine, chutney, curry powder, cumin and tomato puree. Stir into onion mixture and cook over a medium heat for 2-3 minutes. Add chicken and potatoes and cook over a low heat for 5 minutes, or until chicken is tender. Just prior to serving sprinkle with coriander.

205 Calories (855 kilojoules) per serve

Carbohydrate	31.5 g	High
Protein	15.0 g	
Fat	1.0 g	Low
Fibre	4.7 g	Medium

Hot Chicken and Potato Curry

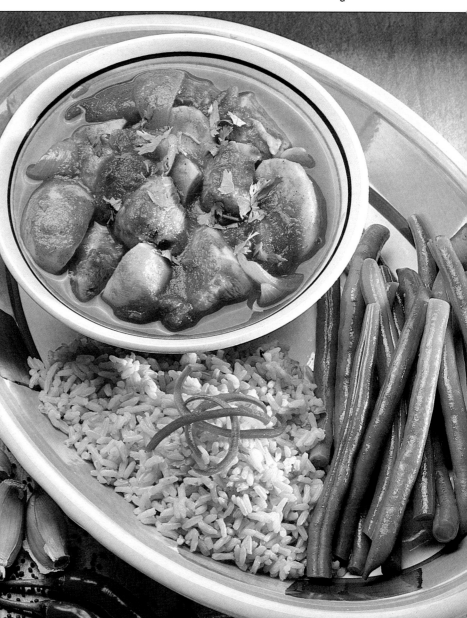

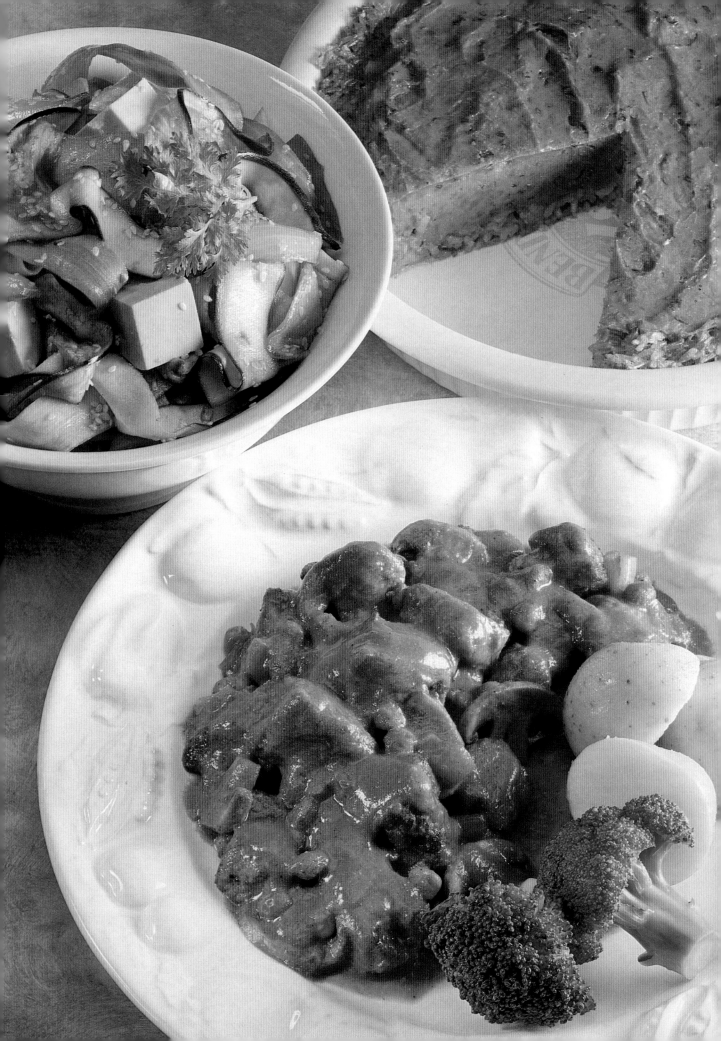

VEAL GOULASH

Serves 4

- ☐ **500 g (1 lb) veal medallions or escalopes**
- ☐ **1 tablespoon paprika**
- ☐ **2 tablespoons plain flour**
- ☐ **¹/₂ teaspoon ground black pepper**
- ☐ **2 teaspoons olive oil**
- ☐ **2 onions, chopped**
- ☐ **2 cloves garlic, crushed**
- ☐ **125 g (4 oz) button mushrooms, sliced**
- ☐ **125 mL (4 fl oz) creamed tomatoes, no-added-salt**
- ☐ **2 tablespoons sweet sherry**
- ☐ **125 mL (4 fl oz) beef stock**
- ☐ **125 g (4 oz) frozen peas**
- ☐ **3 tablespoons low-fat natural yogurt**
- ☐ **2 tablespoons fresh chopped parsley**

1 Trim veal of all visible fat and cut into 2 cm (³/₄ in) pieces. Place paprika, flour and black pepper in a plastic food bag, add veal and shake to coat evenly. Shake off excess flour mixture.

2 Heat oil in a large saucepan and cook veal for 3-4 minutes. Remove veal from pan and set aside. Add onions, garlic and mushrooms and cook for 2-3 minutes, or until onion is soft. Stir in creamed tomatoes, sherry and stock, bring to the boil, then reduce heat and simmer uncovered for 20 minutes.

3 Return veal to pan and stir in peas, and cook over a low heat for 5 minutes or until heated through. Remove pan from heat, stir in yogurt and parsley and serve immediately.

Serving suggestion: For a balanced meal serve with brown rice and a green salad, or vegetables such as pumpkin and beans.

240 Calories (1005 kilojoules) per serve

Carbohydrate	12.0 g	Low
Protein	34.0 g	
Fat	5.0 g	Low
Fibre	3.5 g	Medium

VEGETABLE STIR-FRY

Serves 4

- ☐ **500 g (1 lb) tofu, cut into small cubes**
- ☐ **2 tablespoons reduced-salt soy sauce**
- ☐ **1 red chilli, finely chopped**
- ☐ **1 teaspoon sesame oil**
- ☐ **2 teaspoons honey, warmed**
- ☐ **2 carrots, peeled**
- ☐ **2 courgettes**
- ☐ **1 small aubergine**
- ☐ **1 parsnip**
- ☐ **2 teaspoons polyunsaturated oil**
- ☐ **2 onions, cut into eighths**
- ☐ **2 tablespoons sesame seeds**

1 Place tofu, soy sauce, chilli, sesame oil and honey in a bowl and set aside to marinate for 15-20 minutes.

2 Peel strips from carrots, courgettes, aubergine and parsnip, using a wide-bladed vegetable peeler, then cut into ribbons using a small sharp knife. Set aside.

3 Heat oil in a wok or frying pan and stir-fry onions for 3 minutes or until soft. Add carrots, courgettes, aubergine, parsnip and sesame seeds, and stir-fry for 6-8 minutes, or until vegetables are tender crisp.

4 Stir tofu and marinade into pan and toss gently for 2 minutes, or until tofu is heated through.

205 Calories (860 kilojoules) per serve

Carbohydrate	11.0 g	Low
Protein	13.0 g	
Fat	12.0 g	High
Fibre	4.1 g	Medium

RICE PIE

Serves 4
Oven temperature 180°C, 350°F, Gas 4

- ☐ **220 g (7 oz) brown rice, cooked**
- ☐ **2 egg whites**
- ☐ **2 tablespoons grated fresh Parmesan cheese**
- ☐ **¹/₄ teaspoon chilli powder**

SWEET POTATO FILLING
- ☐ **750 g (1¹/₂ lb) sweet potato or potato, peeled, cooked and mashed**
- ☐ **2 eggs, lightly beaten**
- ☐ **¹/₂ teaspoon ground nutmeg**
- ☐ **¹/₂ teaspoon ground cumin**
- ☐ **2 tablespoons snipped fresh chives**

1 Place rice, egg whites, Parmesan cheese and chilli powder in a bowl and mix to combine. Press mixture into a lightly greased 20 cm (8 in) pie plate.

2 To make filling, place sweet potato, egg, nutmeg, cumin and chives in a bowl and mix to combine. Spoon over rice base and bake for 20-25 minutes, or until filling is firm.

Serving suggestion: Can be served hot, warm or cold. With its high carbohydrate and low fat content, small slices of this pie make an ideal snack.

270 Calories (1145 kilojoules) per serve

Carbohydrate	47.0 g	High
Protein	10.0 g	
Fat	5.0 g	Low
Fibre	7.7 g	High

ARE CARBOHYDRATES FATTENING?

Carbohydrate foods, particularly bread and potatoes have long had the reputation for making people fat. Carbohydrates actually contain less energy than fats and are less readily converted to fat in the body. Whilst excessive carbohydrate intake will eventually increase weight, fats will do it more readily. In other words, fats are more fattening than carbohydrates.

- 1 g fat = 37 kJ (9 Cals)
- 1 g carbohydrate = 16 kJ (4 Cals)

Rice Pie, Vegetable Stir-Fry, Veal Goulash

TOMATO AND SPINACH MEAT PIZZA

Serves 6
Oven temperature 180°C, 350°F, Gas 4

- [ ] **185 g (6 oz) cracked wheat soaked in 500 mL (16 fl oz) hot water for 10-15 minutes**
- [ ] **1 onion, chopped**
- [ ] **1 clove garlic, crushed**
- [ ] **500 g (1 lb) lean minced lamb**
- [ ] **1/2 teaspoon mixed herbs**
- [ ] **1 tablespoon lemon juice**
- [ ] **1 tablespoon chopped fresh mint**
- [ ] **1/2 teaspoon chilli powder**

TOMATO AND HUMMUS TOPPING
- [ ] **220 g (7 oz) hummus**
- [ ] **2 tomatoes, sliced**
- [ ] **8 spinach leaves, blanched and chopped**
- [ ] **3 tablespoons pine nuts**
- [ ] **4 tablespoons grated low-fat cheddar cheese**

1 Drain cracked wheat and set aside. Cook onion and garlic in a nonstick frying pan for 3 minutes or until onion is soft. Transfer cracked wheat and onion mixture to a bowl and combine with lamb, mixed herbs, lemon juice, mint and chilli powder.

2 Press meat mixture into a 32 cm (12 1/2 in) pizza tray and cook for 20 minutes or until base is firm. Drain off any juices.

3 To make topping, spread meat pizza base with hummus then top with tomato slices and spinach. Sprinkle with pine nuts and cheese. Cook under a preheated grill for 3-4 minutes or until cheese melts.

Serving suggestion: Cut pizza into wedges and serve with crusty bread and a salad.

360 Calories (1515 kilojoules) per serve

Carbohydrate	*25.0 g*	*Low*
Protein	*27.0 g*	
Fat	*17.0 g*	*High*
Fibre	*2.0 g*	*Medium*

Below: Tomato and Spinach Meat Pizza
Right: Speedy Salmon Rissoles

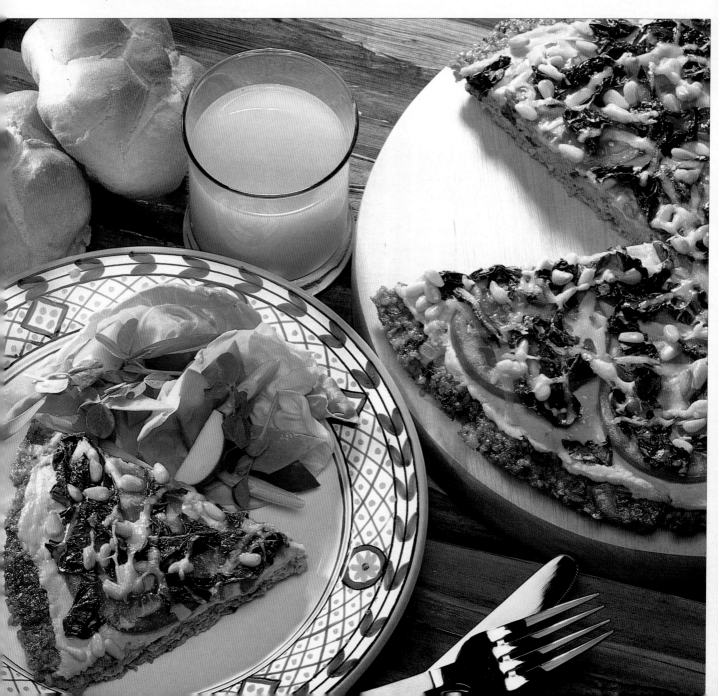

Takeaway tucker

Fast foods may be fast to eat but they definitely do not make you fast on the athletic field!

Unfortunately, fast food is generally high in fat, cholesterol and salt. Active people with hearty appetites can eat large quantities of fast food without getting full, as there is usually little complex carbohydrate or fibre to fill them up. The occasional indulgence is not a problem, providing it is not a precompetition meal. Follow these guidelines for the best fast food and restaurant choices.

THE TAKEAWAY BAR

Do order: Plain hamburgers with salad, steak sandwiches, barbecue chicken (skin removed), thick crust pizza (no extra cheese), sandwiches, rolls, pitta bread (preferably wholemeal), jacket potatoes with topping (but no sour cream), fruit, fruit salads, dried fruit, low-fat yogurts, juices, plain mineral water, plain scones, fruit buns, wholemeal muffins.

Best avoided: French fries, any battered food such as chicken, fish or sausages, crumbed meats, pies, sausage rolls, fatty meats such as salami, cream cakes or desserts, confectionery or crisps.

ITALIAN

Do order: Vegetable antipasto, minestrone or vegetable soup, grissini bread sticks, crusty bread, calamari salad, prosciutto and melon, ravioli, tortellini, spaghetti, fettuccine or other pasta with any of these sauces – napolitana (tomato), marinara (seafood), bolognaise (meat), primavera (vegetable), putanesca (tomato, vegetable and olives) – chicken cacciatore, grilled garlic chicken, veal scallopini, osso bucco, pizza with thick crust (avoid too much cheese), gelato and fresh fruits.

Best avoided: Garlic or herb bread, salami, pepperoni, any fried food, cannelloni, lasagne, pasta with cream sauces, saltimbocca (veal with ham and cheese), zabaglione and cassata.

CHINESE

Do order: Clear short soups with or without wontons or dumplings, crab and corn soup, steamed dim sims or wontons, pork and lettuce rolls, satay prawns, steamed fish with black bean sauce, steamed rice, combination vegetables, stir-fry dishes with lean meat, chicken or pork, chow mein dishes, chop suey dishes, Mongolian hot pot, Chinese tea and lychees.

Best avoided: Any deep-fried foods, crisp skin chicken, chicken in lemon sauce, sweet and sour dishes, fried rice, fried noodles, Peking duck, pork spare ribs, deep-fried whole fish and chicken wings.

MIDDLE EASTERN

Do order: Hummus, aubergine dip, flatbread, pitta bread, tabbouleh, kafta, shish kebabs, souvlaki, shawarma or doner kebab, kibbi, rice-stuffed marrow or courgettes, yogurt and cucumber dip.

Best avoided: Falafel, spicy sausages, baklava, bread with oil or melted butter.

7 fat savers

- Ask for little or no butter on sandwiches and rolls.
- Ask for extra plain bread (no butter).
- Ask for extra salad (without dressing).
- Ask for food to be grilled not pan- or deep-fried.
- Order extra steamed vegetables and rice.
- Remove skin from poultry before eating.
- Avoid dishes with cream sauces.

Fat finder

Low-fat diets assist active people to maintain their lean physique.

Most Western diets contain too much fat. Since fats have more calories (kilojoules) than any other nutrient, excessive intake may lead to obesity. Fat should ideally provide less than 30 per cent of your daily energy. Athletes range from being too blase to obsessive about fat intake; neither extreme is good.

TYPES OF FAT

Triglycerides and cholesterol are the two main groups of fat in our diet. Intake of both needs to be kept to a minimum.

● **Cholesterol:** This is found in foods such as liver, kidney, egg yolk, butter and cheese etc. Excessive cholesterol intake has been linked with coronary heart disease, but it is now regarded to be less important than the excessive intake of saturated fat.

There are three main types of triglycerides:

● **Saturated:** These include butter, lard, cheese, fat on meat, coconut, whole milk etc. It should be noted that an excess of saturated fat is linked with elevated blood cholesterol and coronary heart disease. Replacing this fat with either mono-unsaturated or polyunsaturated fats is recommended.

● **Mono-unsaturated:** These include olive, peanut or canola oil and avocado.

● **Polyunsaturated:** These include sunflower, safflower, fish, fish oils and polyunsaturated margarine.

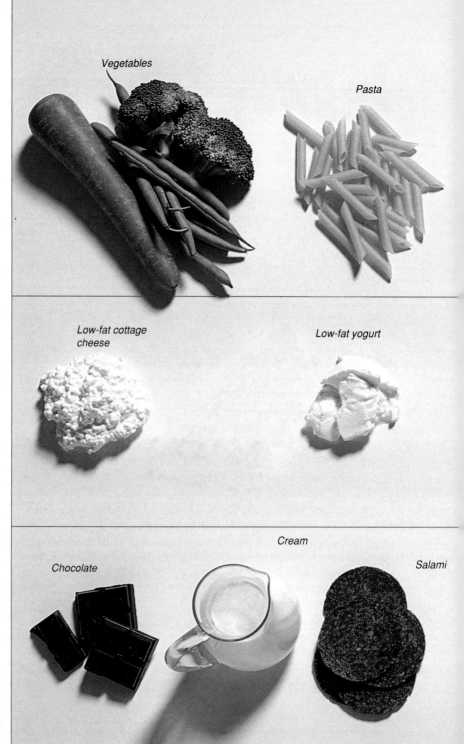

Vegetables

Pasta

Low-fat cottage cheese

Low-fat yogurt

Chocolate

Cream

Salami

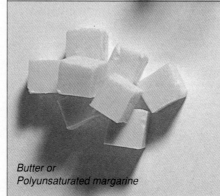

Butter or Polyunsaturated margarine

THE HIDDEN OPPONENT

In practical terms it is easy to cut down on visible fat, such as spreads, the fat on meat or skin on chicken, salad dressings or that extra helping of cream. However, to successfully cut fat we need to be aware of the hidden fats in food. The fat finder will assist you to recognise some of these sources.

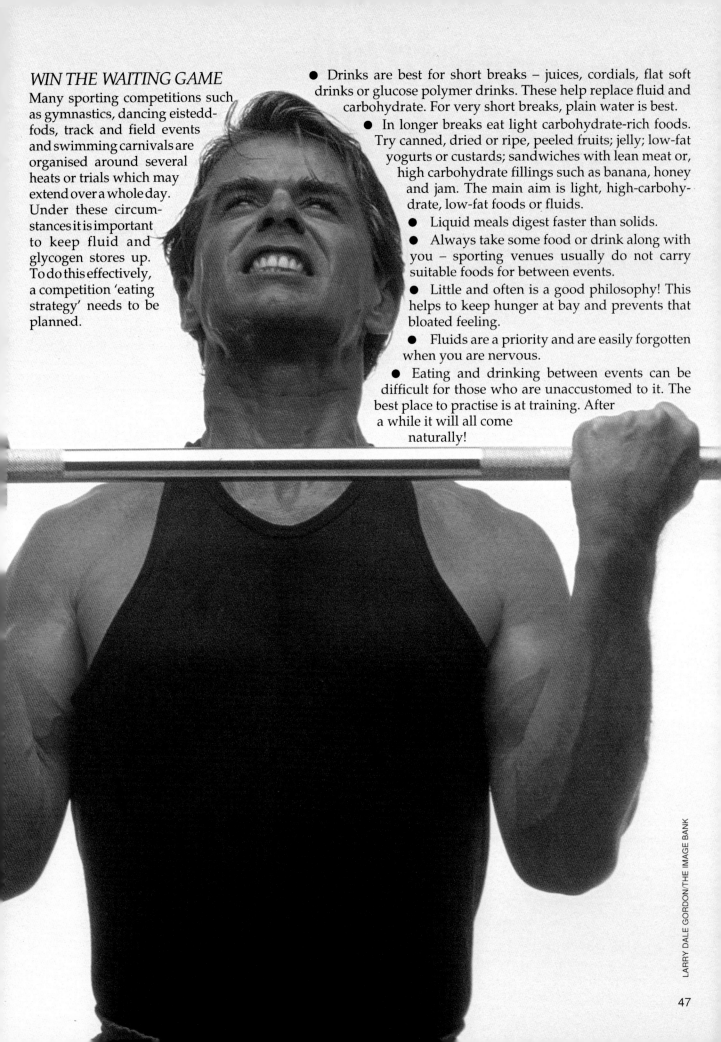

WIN THE WAITING GAME

Many sporting competitions such as gymnastics, dancing eisteddfods, track and field events and swimming carnivals are organised around several heats or trials which may extend over a whole day. Under these circumstances it is important to keep fluid and glycogen stores up. To do this effectively, a competition 'eating strategy' needs to be planned.

● Drinks are best for short breaks – juices, cordials, flat soft drinks or glucose polymer drinks. These help replace fluid and carbohydrate. For very short breaks, plain water is best.

● In longer breaks eat light carbohydrate-rich foods. Try canned, dried or ripe, peeled fruits; jelly; low-fat yogurts or custards; sandwiches with lean meat or, high carbohydrate fillings such as banana, honey and jam. The main aim is light, high-carbohydrate, low-fat foods or fluids.

● Liquid meals digest faster than solids.

● Always take some food or drink along with you – sporting venues usually do not carry suitable foods for between events.

● Little and often is a good philosophy! This helps to keep hunger at bay and prevents that bloated feeling.

● Fluids are a priority and are easily forgotten when you are nervous.

● Eating and drinking between events can be difficult for those who are unaccustomed to it. The best place to practise is at training. After a while it will all come naturally!

Precompetition menu planner

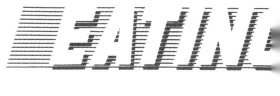

Make the most of what you eat when it's a week before you compete. Use this seven day menu planner as a guide.

Day 1

Breakfast
Fruit juice
Rolled oats with low-fat milk
Peaches and Cream Muffins (p. 8)

Lunch
Golden Soup (p. 26)
Wholemeal bread roll spread thinly with polyunsaturated margarine, reduced-fat spread or butter
Cheesy Bean Potatoes (p. 31)
Green salad
Fresh fruit
Natural mineral water

Dinner
Honey Beef (p. 66)
Steamed brown rice
Green salad with Oriental Dressing (p. 28)
Wholemeal bread roll spread thinly with polyunsaturated margarine, reduced-fat spread or butter
Tropical Crepes (p. 72)

Snacks
1 piece fresh fruit
200 g carton low-fat yogurt
1 No Fussin' Muffin (p. 38)
1 Smashing Smoothie (p. 50)

Day 2

Breakfast
$^1/_2$ small rock melon sprinkled with sultanas
Vegetable Hash Browns (p. 10)
2 slices wholemeal toast or bread spread thinly with polyunsaturated margarine, reduced-fat spread or butter
'Shake it up' milkshake (p. 51)

Lunch
Pasta Vegetable Medley (p. 61)
1 cup fruit salad
200 g carton low-fat yogurt
Fruit juice

Dinner
Quick Cutlet Crumble (p. 64)
Boiled new potatoes (2 small)
Green salad with Fast French Dressing (p. 28)
Wholemeal bread roll spread thinly with polyunsaturated margarine, reduced-fat spread or butter
Fresh fruit
Fruit juice

Snacks
2 slices raisin toast spread thinly with polyunsaturated margarine, reduced-fat spread or butter
2 pieces fresh fruit or 2 glasses fruit juice

Day 3

Breakfast
Fruit juice
1 cup fresh fruit salad topped with low-fat yogurt and sprinkled with sultanas
Spring Omelette (p. 8)
2 slices wholemeal toast or bread spread thinly with polyunsaturated margarine, reduced-fat spread or butter

Lunch
Rice Pie (p. 33)
Green salad with Fast French Dressing (p. 28)
2 pieces fresh fruit
Natural mineral water

Dinner
Pork Fillets with Red Wine Sauce (p. 26)
Steamed new potatoes (2 small)
Generous servings of your favourite steamed vegetables
Wholemeal bread roll spread thinly with polyunsaturated margarine, reduced-fat spread or butter
Fruity Strudel (p. 70)
Fruit juice

Snacks
3 Wholemeal Scones with Strawberry Spread (p. 55)
1 Smashing Smoothie (p. 50)
Fruit juice

Day 4

Breakfast
Fruit juice
Melon Cups with Yogurt Dressing (p. 9)
Wholegrain breakfast cereal with low-fat milk
2 wholemeal crumpets spread thinly with polyunsaturated margarine, reduced-fat spread or butter then topped with a drizzle of honey

---

SERVING SIZES		
Rice, cooked .... 185 g (6 oz)		Rolled oats, cooked .... 250 g (8 oz)
Fruit juice .... 250 mL (8 fl oz)		Wholegrain cereal ..... 30-60 g (1-2 oz)

Lunch
Tasty Hawaiian Pockets (p. 10)
Fresh fruit
Pineapple Punch (p. 51)

Dinner
Mexican Chilli Pasta (p. 66)
Green salad with Tangy Cucumber Dressing (p. 29)
Wholemeal bread roll spread thinly with polyunsaturated margarine, reduced-fat spread or butter
Fresh fruit
Fruit spritzer (fruit juice and natural mineral water)

Snacks
Speedy Date Slice (p. 40)
200 g (6^1/2 oz) carton natural low-fat yogurt mixed with dried fruit of your choice
1 piece fresh fruit

Day
5

Breakfast
Large fruit juice
Fruity Porridge (p. 10) with low-fat milk and a dollop of natural low-fat yogurt drizzled with honey
Fresh fruit

Lunch
Vegetarian Pan Pizza (p. 22)
Green salad with Island Hopping Dressing (p. 29)
Wholemeal bread roll spread thinly with polyunsaturated margarine, reduced-fat spread or butter
Hot Fruit Salad (p. 68)
Fruit juice

Dinner
Hot Chicken and Potato Curry (p. 31)
Steamed vegetables of your choice
Wholemeal bread roll spread thinly with polyunsaturated margarine, reduced-fat spread or butter

Complementary stewed fruit with Apricot Bread Pudding (p. 71)
Natural mineral water

Snacks
Pineapple Punch (p. 51)
2 slices wholemeal toast with a scrape of polyunsaturated margarine, reduced-fat spread or butter and topped with jam
1 piece fresh fruit

Day
6

Breakfast
Fruit juice
Mighty Muesli with low-fat milk (p. 6)
2 slices wholemeal toast topped with honey mashed banana and cinnamon

Lunch
Multi-Layered bread loaf (p. 15)
Fresh fruit
Fruit juice

Dinner
Vegetable and Lentil Soup (p. 62)
Wholemeal bread roll spread thinly with polyunsaturated margarine
Vegetable Pilaf (p. 62)
Green salad dressed with lemon vinegar
Summer Pudding (p. 72)
Fruit juice

Snacks
2 Ginger 'n' Fruit Cookies (p. 38)
Melon Marbles (p. 56)
1 Smashing Smoothie (p. 50)

Day
7

Breakfast
Fruit Tango (p. 50)
1 cup fruit salad

MEAL PLANS EXPLAINED

Each daily menu provides approximately 3000 Calories (12,600 kilojoules): 2500 Calories (10,500 kilojoules) from meals, 500 Calories (2100 kilojoules) from snacks. The energy (calorie/kilojoule) level is suitable for active males. For females and those less active, smaller servings and reducing or omitting snacks etc. will help to decrease the energy to the appropriate level. Alternatively, increasing foods such as bread, fruit, juice, rice, pasta will increase the energy and carbohydrate in the daily menu.

The proportion of energy from protein, fat and carbohydrate is approximately 20% protein, 20% fat and 60% carbohydrate for Days 1-3. With a view to increasing glycogen stores for a competition on the morning of Day 7 the proportion of carbohydrate was increased on Days 4-7 to 70%, decreasing protein and fat to 15% each.

Wholegrain cereal with low-fat milk
2 Spicy Pancakes with Banana Yogurt topping (pp. 6-7)

Lunch
Minestrone Soup (p. 24)
Golden Grain Salad (p. 14)
Wholegrain bread roll spread thinly with polyunsaturated margarine, reduced-fat spread or butter
200 g (6^1/2 oz) carton low-fat yogurt
Fresh fruit
Fruit juice

Dinner
Chicken Stir-fry (p. 64)
Boiled noodles (400 g)
Green salad
Creamy Berry Rice (p. 69)
Fruit juice

Snacks
2 slices raisin toast spread thinly with polyunsaturated margarine, reduced-fat spread or butter, topped with honey
1 piece fresh fruit

Dive into a drink

SMASHING SMOOTHIES

Serves 2

- [ ] **2 bananas, peeled and sliced**
- [ ] **200 g (6¹/2 oz) low-fat fruit salad yogurt**
- [ ] **2 tablespoons skimmed milk powder**
- [ ] **375 mL (12 fl oz) skimmed milk**
- [ ] **¹/4 teaspoon ground mixed spice**
- [ ] **fresh mint sprig**

Place bananas, yogurt, skimmed milk powder, skimmed milk and mixed spice in a food processor or blender and process until smooth. Pour into a tall chilled glass and garnish with mint.

Apricot Smoothie: Replace bananas with 250 g (8 oz) diced canned apricot and fruit salad yogurt with low-fat apricot yogurt. Omit mixed spice and add 1 teaspoon finely grated orange rind.

Strawberry Smoothie: Replace bananas with 250 g (8 oz) strawberries washed and hulled, and fruit salad yogurt with low-fat strawberry yogurt. Omit mixed spice.

310 Calories(1300 kilojoules) per serve
Carbohydrate	*60.0 g*	*High*
Protein	*16.5 g*	
Fat	*1.0 g*	*Low*
Fibre	*3.5 g*	*Medium*

(Analysis for basic recipe)

EGG FLIP

Serves 1

- [ ] **250 mL (8 fl oz) skimmed milk**
- [ ] **2 tablespoons skimmed milk powder**
- [ ] **1 egg**
- [ ] **¹/2 teaspoon vanilla essence**
- [ ] **1 tablespoon honey**
- [ ] **pinch ground nutmeg**

Place skimmed milk, skimmed milk powder, egg, vanilla essence and honey in a food processor or blender and process until smooth. Pour into a tall glass and sprinkle with nutmeg.

305 Calories (1275 kilojoules) per serve
Carbohydrate	*44.0 g*	*Medium*
Protein	*21.0 g*	
Fat	*6.0 g*	*Low*
Fibre	*none*	*Low*

FRUIT TANGO

Serves 4

- [ ] **500 mL (16 fl oz) orange juice**
- [ ] **500 mL (16 fl oz) apple juice**
- [ ] **500 mL (16 fl oz) pineapple juice**
- [ ] **pulp of 4 passion fruit**
- [ ] **500 mL (16 fl oz) sparkling mineral water**
- [ ] **3 tablespoons finely chopped fresh mint**
- [ ] **2 trays ice cubes**

Combine orange, apple and pineapple juices, passion fruit pulp, mineral water and mint in a large punch bowl. Chill until ready to serve. Just prior to serving, add ice cubes.

105 Calories (450 kilojoules) per serve
Carbohydrate	*25.0 g*	*High*
Protein	*1.0 g*	
Fat	*neg*	*Low*
Fibre	*2.3 g*	*Medium*

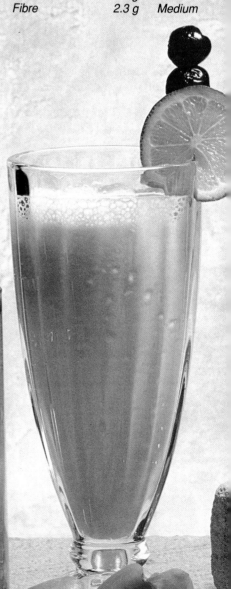

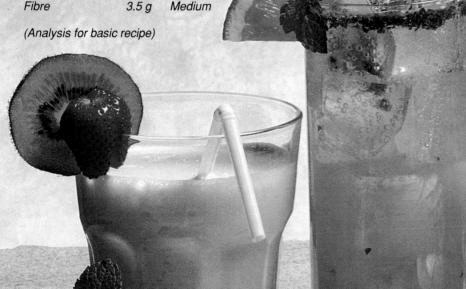

SHAKE IT UP

Serves 1

- ☐ **250 mL (8 fl oz) skimmed milk**
- ☐ **2 tablespoons skimmed milk powder**
- ☐ **¹/₂ teaspoon vanilla essence**
- ☐ **1 tablespoon honey**
- ☐ **1 scoop vanilla ice cream**

Place skimmed milk, skimmed milk powder, vanilla essence, honey and ice cream in a food processor or blender and process until smooth. Pour into a well-chilled tall glass and serve.

310 Calories (1300 kilojoules) per serve

Carbohydrate	55.5 g	High
Protein	16.5 g	
Fat	3.5 g	Low
Fibre	none	Low

From left: Egg Flip, Fruit Tango, Shake It Up, Pineapple Punch, Strawberry Smoothie

PINEAPPLE PUNCH

Serves 1

- ☐ **125 g (4 oz) low-fat natural yogurt**
- ☐ **125 mL (4 fl oz) pineapple juice**
- ☐ **3 tablespoons crushed pineapple**
- ☐ **1 scoop vanilla ice cream**

Place yogurt, pineapple juice, crushed pineapple and ice cream in a food processor or blender and process until smooth. Pour into a tall glass and serve.

275 Calories (1160 kilojoules) per serve

Carbohydrate	52.0 g	High
Protein	9.0 g	
Fat	4.0 g	Low
Fibre	1.2 g	Low

WHAT ABOUT WATER?

Many active people have grown up with the myth that it is detrimental to drink water during exercise.

- ● Fluid replacement is the most vital of all competition strategies, and failure to replace lost fluids can be detrimental to performance and hazardous to health!
- ● In most cases water is the best replacement drink.
- ● Water replacement alone is adequate for short duration or non-endurance events.
- ● Cold or refrigerated water is ideal as it empties most rapidly from the stomach.
- ● In 'ultra' endurance events (longer than three hours) substantial glycogen and salt losses can occur during the competition. Sports (electrolyte replacement) drinks help to replace the carbohydrate and salt along with water.

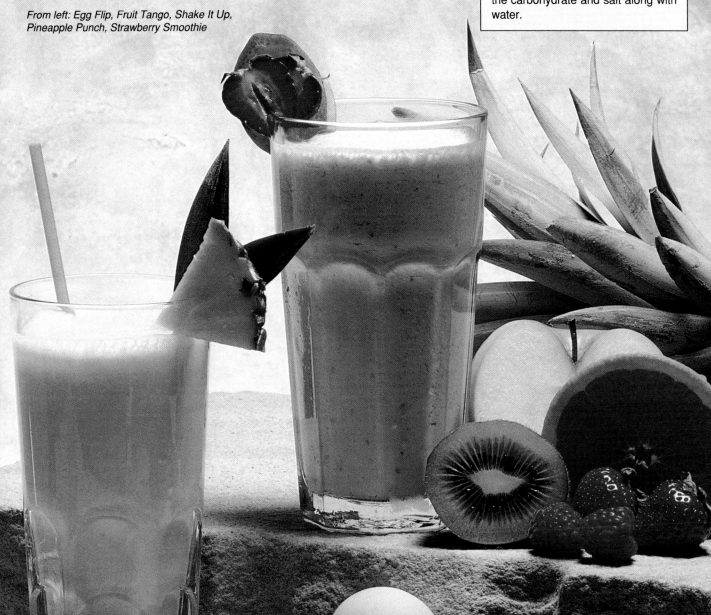

Too hot to trot?

9 ways to keep cool

- During hot weather, exercise at cooler times of the day.
- Gradually acclimatise yourself to weather conditions.
- Wear comfortable clothing that allows you to sweat freely.
- Use a sun screen and a hat to keep the sun's rays at bay in hot weather.
- Avoid exercising when you are unwell.
- Learn to recognise the symptoms of heat stress.
- Drink cool water regularly.
- Do not delay drinking – it is too hard to catch up once dehydration sets in.
- Practise fluid replacement during training.

Exercise increases the body's heat production. Sweating helps to prevent the body from getting too hot!

To sweat, the body must be well hydrated. If dehydration sets in, body temperature rises and heat stress results. In severe cases permanent physical damage or death can occur! Although athletes sweat more effectively and cope with the heat better than untrained people, they can still experience heat stress.

PREVENTING HEAT STRESS

Regular fluid consumption during exercise helps to replace sweat losses, prevent dehydration and heat stress.

The symptoms of heat stress start slowly. Early warning signs include fatigue, headache, feeling hot, dizzy or nauseous. As the condition worsens, disorientation or incoherence occur and sweating may stop all together. At this stage, most people are too confused to stop themselves and event organisers need to step in. Severe heat stress needs urgent medical attention.

SPORTS DRINKS

Controversy continues over the ideal composition of sports (electrolyte replacement) drinks used during exercise. The major concern is the rate at which they empty from the stomach – the more concentrated the drink, the longer it takes to be emptied from the stomach and absorbed into the blood stream. Delayed emptying is considered to jeopardise hydration and slow-emptying drinks can cause nausea during exercise.

Many new sports drinks, available from pharmacies, contain glu-

---

FLUID REPLACEMENT

The amount of fluid needed to balance losses depends on the intensity and duration of exercise as well as the environmental conditions. It is not unusual for elite athletes to sweat more than 1 litre per hour.

To replace fluid loss:

- Consume 150-300 millilitres (5-9 1/2 fluid ounces) of fluid for every 20-30 minutes of strenuous exercise.
- Children and adolescents require 75-200 millilitres (1 1/2-6 1/2 fluid ounces) of fluid over a similar time frame.
- Ideally, an extra 250-500 millilitres (8-16 fluid ounces) of fluid should be taken 20-30 minutes prior to the event.
- Endurance athletes benefit from increasing their fluid intake 24 hours prior to competition.

---

cose polymers which empty almost as rapidly as water from the stomach. The glucose helps to delay fatigue and maintain blood sugar levels during exercise. As a general rule, drinks consumed during exercise should not exceed 10 per cent carbohydrate.

REFUELLING

People competing in endurance events extending 2-3 hours need to replace carbohydrates, as well as fluids during competition. Sports drinks combine hydration with refuelling. Carbohydrate-rich foods, in conjunction with sports drinks, also assist carbohydrate and energy replacement.

Those competing in endurance events are advised to consume about 50 grams of carbohydrate per hour. Each athlete needs to experiment to determine which foods work best for them.

Boning up on calcium

Moderate exercise and an adequate intake of calcium throughout life help to make bones strong and prevent osteoporosis.

Osteoporosis or 'thinning of the bones' occurs in both men and women as they age. However, it is more prevalent in women.

PREVENTING OSTEOPOROSIS
● Exercise generally strengthens bones.
● Some women who train intensely can develop amenorrhoea (absence of menstruation associated with reduced body fat, and/or intense training), a condition which appears to increase the risk of osteoporosis and stress fractures.
● The following are all thought to increase the risk of developing osteoporosis but more research is required to establish their relative importance :
 • family history of osteoporosis
 • inactivity
 • total or partial absence of menstruation
 • inadequate calcium intake
 • excessive intake of protein, salt, alcohol or bran fibre

TREATING OSTEOPOROSIS
● Ensure an adequate calcium intake throughout life. It is preferable that calcium comes from the diet rather than supplements.
● Treatment of osteoporosis may involve use of oestrogen replacement and calcium supplements. These should only be taken under medical supervision.

CALCIUM WITHOUT FAT
Reduced- or low-fat dairy products are an excellent source of calcium. Some milk products have additional calcium added and are therefore higher in calcium than regular milk. Reduced- or low-fat dairy foods are useful for people who need to watch their fat or cholesterol intake or for those who are watching their weight. These dairy foods are fine for children over the age of 2 years but younger children need regular milk to obtain sufficient calories (kilojoules) for growth.

GOOD FOOD SOURCES OF CALCIUM

FOOD	SERVE SIZE	CALCIUM (mg)
Whole milk	250 mL (8 fl oz)	310
Skim milk	250 mL (8 fl oz)	311
Reduced-fat (2%), fortified milk	250 mL (8 fl oz)	374
Natural yogurt	small carton (200 g/6^1/2 oz)	390
Low-fat fruit yogurt	small carton (200 g/6^1/2 oz)	345
Processed cheddar cheese	1 slice (21 g/^{3}/4 oz)	131
Reduced-fat cheddar cheese	1 slice (21 g/^{3}/4 oz)	170
Low-fat cottage cheese	1 tablespoon (20 g/^{3}/4 oz)	15
Reduced-fat ricotta cheese	1 tablespoon (20 g/^{3}/4 oz)	49
Vanilla ice cream	2 scoops (90 g/3 oz)	120
Red salmon	100 g (3^1/2 oz)	225
Sardines (in oil)	100 g (3^1/2 oz)	302
Oysters (raw)	12 oysters	79
Kidney beans	1 cup (170 g/5^1/2 oz) boiled	19
Tofu	100 g (3^1/2 oz)	128
Fortified soy drink	1 cup (250 mL/8 fl oz)	290
Dried apricots	5 halves (20 g/^{3}/4 oz)	23
Sesame seeds	1 tablespoon (10 g/^{1}/3 oz)	13
Almonds	45 g (1^1/2 oz) pack	125

Reprinted with permission. Source: Commonwealth Department of Community Services and Health 1989, NUTTAB Version 89. Food Industry Data and Sanitarium Nutrition Education leaflets, June 1990.

The sports canteen

Many sporting clubs and venues have a canteen, but unfortunately the choices of healthy foods at these canteens are limited.

Serving healthy food in this environment can help to educate children and parents about the correct diet. As a result, many such places are now switching to health-oriented canteens. A little planning can make them just as popular and profitable as their less healthy predecessors. The following should give you some ideas!

CANTEEN GUIDELINES

The canteen can be important as a practical example of nutrition and health.

● Be involved in the development of your children's, or your own, club's policy on what the canteen should provide for lunches and snacks.

● Follow the Healthy Diet Pyramid plan (see page 20), which emphasises foods rich in complex carbohydrate, protein, vitamins and minerals and low in fat, sugar and salt.

● Encourage the sale of low-fat foods such as sandwiches and bread rolls with low-fat fillings, and salad and fruit as an alternative to pies, sausage rolls and fried foods.

● Introduce reduced-fat and low-fat milk drinks, yogurt and cheese.

● Have tasting sessions and special promotions – just like the local supermarket does – to find out which foods are the most popular.

MINI QUICHES

Makes 6
Oven temperature 200°C, 400°F, Gas 6

- ☐ **315 g (10 oz) ready-rolled or prepared wholemeal shortcrust pastry, thawed**
- ☐ **1 onion, finely chopped**
- ☐ **220 g (7 oz) canned salmon, no-added-salt, drained and flaked**
- ☐ **2 eggs, lightly beaten**
- ☐ **185 mL (6 fl oz) skimmed milk**
- ☐ **1/4 teaspoon ground nutmeg**
- ☐ **2 teaspoons chopped fresh dill**
- ☐ **freshly ground black pepper**
- ☐ **60 g (2 oz) grated reduced-fat cheddar cheese**
- ☐ **1 tablespoon snipped fresh chives**

1   Line six 8 cm (3³/₄ in) flan dishes with pastry. Heat a nonstick frying pan and cook onion for 4-5 minutes or until soft. Divide onion into four portions and spread over base of flans, then top with salmon.

2   Combine eggs, milk, nutmeg, dill and black pepper to taste. Pour into flans, sprinkle with cheese and chives and bake for 20 minutes or until filling is firm.

Spinach and Ham Quiches: Boil, steam or microwave 100 g (3 oz) chopped spinach until tender. Divide into four portions and spread over base of flans. Divide 100 g (3 oz) chopped reduced-fat-and-salt ham and 3 tablespoons finely chopped red pepper between flans, then pour over egg mixture, top with cheese and chives and bake for 20 minutes.

300 Calories (1255 kilojoules) per serve

Carbohydrate	*20.0 g*	*Low*
Protein	*17.0 g*	
Fat	*18.0 g*	*High*
Fibre	*0.5 g*	*Low*

Mini Quiches, Tropical Freezers (page 56), Wholemeal Scones with Strawberry Spread

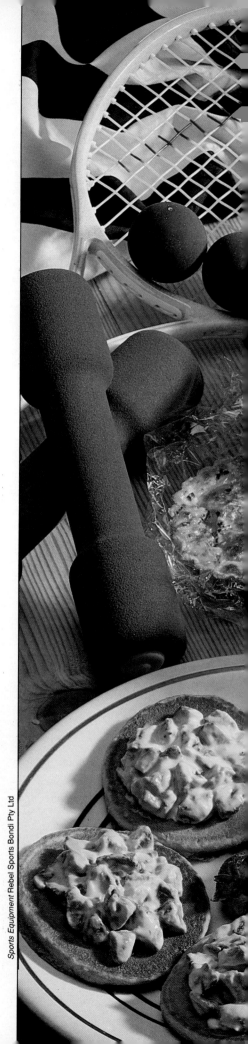

Sports Equipment Rebel Sports Bondi Pty Ltd

54

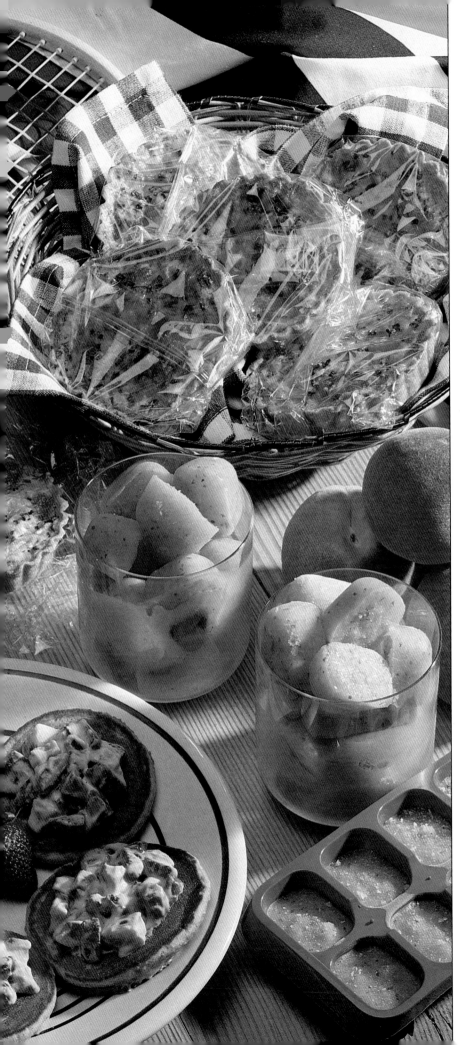

WHOLEMEAL SCONES WITH STRAWBERRY SPREAD

Makes 12 scones

SCONES
- ☐ **185 mL (6 fl oz) skimmed milk**
- ☐ **2 teaspoons polyunsaturated oil**
- ☐ **1 teaspoon lemon juice**
- ☐ **1 egg**
- ☐ **2 tablespoons honey**
- ☐ **155 g (5 oz) wholemeal self-raising flour sifted with 1 teaspoon ground cinnamon and husks returned**
- ☐ **2 teaspoons polyunsaturated margarine**

STRAWBERRY SPREAD
- ☐ **3 tablespoons ricotta cheese**
- ☐ **1 tablespoon low-fat natural yogurt**
- ☐ **2 teaspoons honey**
- ☐ **250 g (8 oz) strawberries, hulled and chopped**

1 To make scones, place skimmed milk, oil, lemon juice, egg and honey in a food processor or blender and process to combine. Add flour mixture and process until smooth.

2 Melt margarine in a nonstick frying pan. Drop a tablespoon of mixture at a time into pan and cook over a medium heat until golden brown on each side.

3 To make spread, place ricotta cheese, yogurt and honey in a food processor or blender and process until smooth. Transfer ricotta mixture to a bowl and fold in strawberries. Cover and chill until ready to use.

Serving suggestion: Top scones with spread and serve. These scones are also delicious served plain.

Variation: Replace strawberries with 2 chopped bananas and add a $^1/_2$ teaspoon nutmeg to the spread.

80 Calories (340 kilojoules) per serve

Carbohydrate	11.0 g	*Medium*
Protein	3.0 g	
Fat	3.0 g	*Medium*
Fibre	1.1 g	*Low*

(Analysis for basic recipe)

TROPICAL FREEZERS

Makes 50

- ☐ **440 g (14 oz) canned crushed pineapple**
- ☐ **2 mangoes, flesh peeled and cut into slices**
- ☐ **1 banana, sliced**
- ☐ **1 tablespoon finely chopped fresh mint**

1   Place pineapple, mangoes, banana and mint in a food processor or blender and process until smooth. Pour mixture into ice cube trays and freeze until firm.
2   Turn fruit freezers out into cups. Eat with fingers.

Strawberry and Watermelon Freezers: Replace pineapple, mangoes and banana with 250 g (8 oz) washed and hulled strawberries and 1/4 watermelon, seeds removed and chopped. Omit mint.

68 Calories (282 kilojoules) per serve

Carbohydrate	*16.0 g*	*High*
Protein	*1.0 g*	
Fat	*neg*	*Low*
Fibre	*13.7 g*	*Low*

(Analysis for basic recipe)

MELON MARBLES

Makes 12

- ☐ **1/2 cantaloupe melon, seeded**
- ☐ **1/2 honeydew melon, seeded**
- ☐ **1/4 watermelon, seeded**
- ☐ **2 teaspoons lemon juice**
- ☐ **1 teaspoon honey**
- ☐ **pulp of 2 passion fruit**

1   Make melon balls from cantaloupe melon, honeydew melon and watermelon, using a melon baller. Combine lemon juice, honey and passion fruit pulp in a bowl. Add melon balls and toss to coat.
2   Thread melon balls alternately onto 12 wooden skewers and refrigerate.

45 Calories (180 kilojoules) per serve

Carbohydrate	*9.0 g*	*High*
Protein	*neg*	
Fat	*neg*	*Low*
Fibre	*1.7 g*	*Low*

OTHER CANTEEN FOODS

Throughout this book you will find recipes that are suitable for a sports canteen. Try serving some of the following:
- ● Multi-Layered Bread Loaf (page 15)
- ● Health Club Sandwiches (page 17)
- ● Vegetable and Salad Roll-Ups (page 19)
- ● Quick and Easy Quiche (page 26)
- ● No Fussin' Muffins (page 38)
- ● Ginger 'n' Fruit Cookies (page 38)
- ● Wholehearted Rockcakes (page 40)
- ● Speedy Date Slice (page 40)
- ● Muesli Slice (page 40)
- ● Oaty Biscuits (page 40)
- ● Any of the drinks from the section Dive into a Drink (pages 50-51)

CRICKET WICKETS

Makes 25
Oven temperature 180°C, 350°F, Gas 4

- ☐ **4 potatoes, cooked and mashed**
- ☐ **1 tablespoon skimmed milk powder**
- ☐ **1 tablespoon chopped fresh parsley**
- ☐ **pinch cayenne pepper**
- ☐ **15 g (1/2 oz) polyunsaturated margarine, melted**
- ☐ **3 tablespoons grated Parmesan cheese**

1   Combine mashed potato with skimmed milk powder, parsley, cayenne pepper and margarine.
2   Spoon mixture into a piping bag fitted with a large star nozzle, and pipe 6 cm (2 1/2 in) lengths of mixture onto a greased and lined baking tray. Sprinkle with Parmesan cheese and bake for 20 minutes or until golden.

20 Calories (85 kilojoules) per serve

Carbohydrate	*2.0 g*	*Low*
Protein	*1.0 g*	
Fat	*1.0 g*	*High*
Fibre	*neg*	*Low*

TOASTIES

Makes 1 sandwich

- ☐ **2 slices wholemeal bread**
- ☐ **7 g (1/4 oz) polyunsaturated margarine**

CHOOSE FROM THE FOLLOWING FILLINGS:
- ☐ **1 egg, pan-cooked without fat in a nonstick frying pan**
- ☐ **1 tablespoon snipped fresh chives**
- ☐ **1 slice lean ham, reduced-fat-and-salt**
- ☐ **1 slice cheddar cheese, reduced-fat- and-salt**
- ☐ **1 canned pineapple ring, drained**
- ☐ **3 tablespoons canned baked beans, no-added-salt**
- ☐ **1 tablespoon cottage cheese**
- ☐ **2 slices tomato**

1   Lightly spread outside of bread with margarine.
2   Place filling of your choice on inside of one slice of bread, top with another slice and cook in a sandwich maker for 2-3 minutes, or until golden on outside.

195 Calories (810 kilojoules) per serve

Carbohydrate	*26.0 g*	*Medium*
Protein	*12.0 g*	
Fat	*4.5 g*	*Medium*
Fibre	*5.0 g*	*Medium*

(Analysis for ham and pineapple combination)

Toasties, Melon Marbles, Cricket Wickets

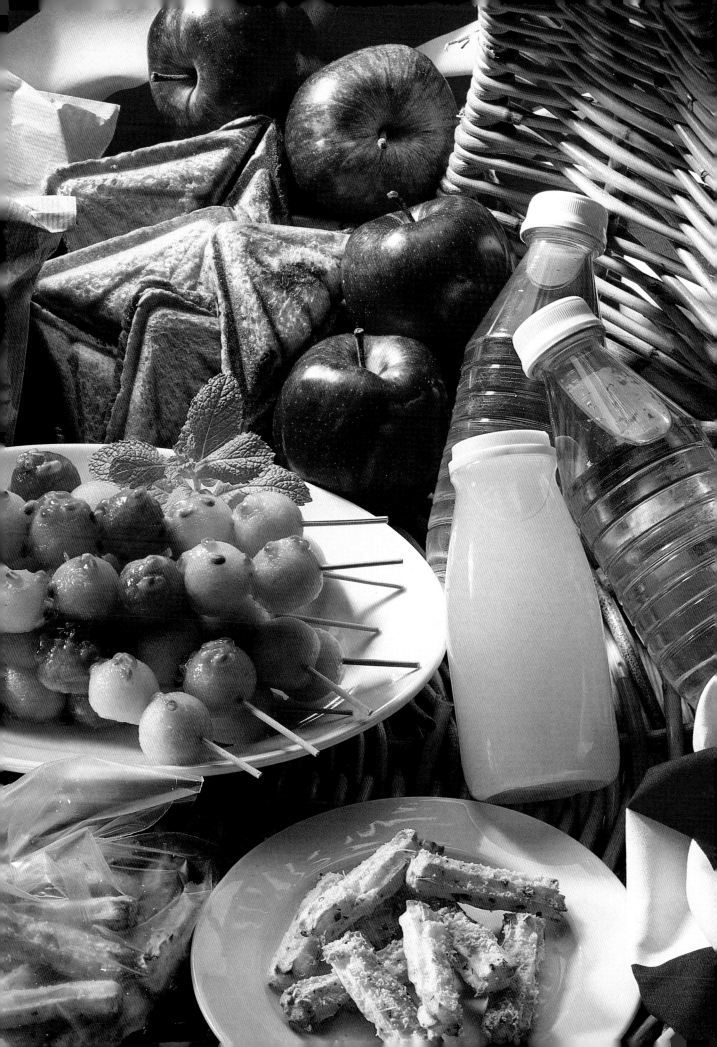

Recipe for recovery

Replacing fluids and glycogen after competition is essential, but often forgotten amidst the celebrations or commiserations.

Drinking liberal amounts of fluid, particularly those rich in carbohydrate (such as fruit juices, soft drinks, cordials and glucose polymers), and following this with a carbohydrate-rich meal, is recommended. Post-competition headaches and muscle cramps are signs that fluids may not have been adequately replaced. Failure to replace carbohydrate will result in fatigue or lethargy in training over the days following competition.

Follow this recipe to assist your recovery after exercise.

RECIPE FOR RECOVERY

☐ **Carbohydrate-based drinks such as fruit juices, cordials, soft drinks, glucose polymer drinks**
☐ **Carbohydrate-rich foods such as bread, rice or pasta, potato and dried peas and beans, fruit and breakfast cereal**
☐ **Water in liberal quantities**
☐ **Minimal to no alcohol**

1 Immediately after exercise, replace lost fluids and glycogen with carbohydrate-based drinks.

2 Evaluate your fluid replacement strategy regularly by measuring your body weight immediately before and after exercise. Every kilogram (pound) lost represents 1 litre ($1^3/4$ pints) of water. Divide the amount lost by your bodyweight and multiply it by 100 to get the percentage lost. Losses greater than 2 per cent affect performance and losses of 5 per cent are dangerous.

3 Passing urine fairly soon after exercise is a good sign that you are fairly well hydrated. If urination is delayed then you need to intensify drinking. Post-exercise headaches or muscle cramps are further side effects of dehydration.

4 The meal taken after exercise needs to be high in carbohydrate.

5 Alcohol consumption after exercise is common, especially in team sports. The main problem with alcohol is its diuretic (dehydrating) properties, which can slow down rehydration. If alcohol is consumed it should be taken only after liberal quantities of non-alcoholic fluids and is best taken with food.

6 Beverages containing caffeine can have a similar diuretic action and excessive consumption is not recommended.

7 After strenuous competitions most people benefit from a lighter training schedule, especially if substantial dehydration has occurred.

WHAT IS A STANDARD DRINK?

ONE STANDARD DRINK

= Low alcohol beer
2 x 280 mL (9 fl oz)

= Ordinary beer
280 mL (9 fl oz)

= Table wine
125 mL (4 fl oz)

= Fortified wine
60 mL (2 fl oz)

= Spirits
30 mL (1 fl oz)

Recommendations for safe alcohol consumption are:
Women: Up to 1-2 standard drinks 4-5 times a week.
Men: Up to 3-4 standard drinks 4-5 times a week.

Safety first

Prevention is better than cure. Follow these simple rules to ensure that you stay injury free.

Starting out: If you are over 35 or have known risk factors, make sure you have a medical check up before starting exercise.

Equipment: The most important areas needing protection are your head and eyes. Use all the protective equipment allowed by the rules (especially helmets). Make sure protective equipment fits properly and is kept in good repair.

Technique: Good technique will help prevent injury – you may need the advice of a coach to help improve your technique.

Overtraining: It is great to be enthusiastic but do not do too much, too soon. When starting out, do not do more than two sessions a week. Each session should be at least two days apart. Gradually increase the number of sessions you do. Muscle soreness that lasts longer than a day means you are overdoing it.

Warm-up: This gradually gets the heart, lungs, muscles and joints ready for exercise. It should involve 5-10 minutes of general aerobic activity, for example jogging on the spot. Stretch the main muscle groups to be used in the sport and practise skills to be performed during the game.

Stretching tips: Stretch each muscle at least twice before exercise and once after exercise. Do not bounce or stretch rapidly. Do not hold your breath while stretching. Hold each stretch 30 to 60 seconds.

Cool-down: This allows the body's systems to gradually slow down. To cool down do the same activities as you did for warming-up but in the reverse order.

Clothing and environment: In hot, humid weather wear loose-fitting clothes that allow airflow over the skin for efficient cooling. Decrease how hard you exercise, and exercise during the coolest part of the day. In cold conditions wear layers of dry, warm clothing to trap body heat. Cover your head, face and hands to avoid heat loss from these areas and make sure that you warm-up properly.

DID YOU KNOW?

Early and effective treatment of a sprained ankle can halve the recovery time.

Priced right

Use the priced principle to treat sprains and strains immediately.

P revent further injury.

R est.

I ce reduces pain, swelling and muscle spasm.

C ompression. Apply a firm wide bandage over the injured part (the bandage must also extend above and below the injury).

E levation. Raise the injured part above the level of the heart.

D iagnosis. Go to a qualified professional, such as a doctor or physiotherapist.

THE RIGHT SPORTS SHOE

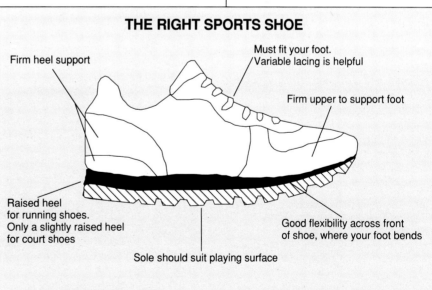

Firm heel support

Must fit your foot. Variable lacing is helpful

Firm upper to support foot

Raised heel for running shoes. Only a slightly raised heel for court shoes

Sole should suit playing surface

Good flexibility across front of shoe, where your foot bends

- If you have problems with your feet, ask for the professional advice of a chiropodist or a physiotherapist.
- Cross-training shoes are good all-round sports shoes.

Family food in a flash

GNOCCHI WITH HERB SAUCE

Serves 4

- [ ] **750 g (1¹/₂ lb) gnocchi**

FRESH HERB SAUCE
- [ ] **4 tablespoons roughly chopped fresh parsley**
- [ ] **4 tablespoons roughly chopped fresh coriander**
- [ ] **4 tablespoons roughly chopped fresh basil**
- [ ] **2 tablespoons pine nuts**
- [ ] **1 tablespoon grated fresh Parmesan cheese**
- [ ] **1 tablespoon reduced-fat mayonnaise**
- [ ] **1 tablespoon vegetable stock**
- [ ] **freshly ground black pepper**

1   Cook gnocchi in a large saucepan of boiling water following packet directions. Drain and set aside to keep warm.

2   To make sauce, place parsley, coriander, basil, pine nuts and Parmesan cheese in a food processor or blender and process until combined. Add mayonnaise and vegetable stock and process until combined. Season to taste with black pepper.

Serving suggestion: Spoon herb sauce over gnocchi and serve immediately. Accompany with a green vegetable or a salad and wholemeal bread rolls.

240 Calories (1015 kilojoules) per serve

Carbohydrate	29.0 g	Medium
Protein	11.0 g	
Fat	9.0 g	Medium
Fibre	2.3 g	Medium

CHILLI TACOS

Serves 4
Oven temperature 180°C, 350°F, Gas 4

- [ ] **8 taco shells**
- [ ] **60 g (2 oz) watercress**
- [ ] **250 g (8 oz) cherry tomatoes, sliced**
- [ ] **90 g (3 oz) grated cheddar cheese, reduced-fat-and-salt**

CHILLI MINCE FILLING
- [ ] **500 g (1 lb) lean minced beef**
- [ ] **1 large onion, chopped**
- [ ] **2 cloves garlic, crushed**
- [ ] **1 teaspoon ground cumin**
- [ ] **1 tablespoon chilli sauce**
- [ ] **125 mL (4 fl oz) creamed tomatoes, no-added-salt**
- [ ] **250 g (8 oz) canned peeled tomatoes, no-added-salt, drained and chopped**

1   To make filling, heat a nonstick frying pan and cook mince, onion and garlic over a medium heat for 5-6 minutes. Stir in cumin, chilli sauce, creamed tomatoes and tomatoes, bring to the boil, then reduce heat and simmer for 10 minutes, or until most of the liquid has evaporated.

2   Place taco shells on an oven tray and warm in oven for 5 minutes. Fill shells with filling, top with watercress, tomato slices and cheese.

Serving suggestion: Tacos make a quick and tasty meal served with savoury rice and a mixed green salad.

355 Calories (1480 kilojoules) per serve

Carbohydrate	17.0 g	Low
Protein	38.0 g	
Fat	15.0 g	High
Fibre	4.5 g	Medium

Chilli Tacos, Pasta Vegetable Medley, Gnocchi with Herb Sauce

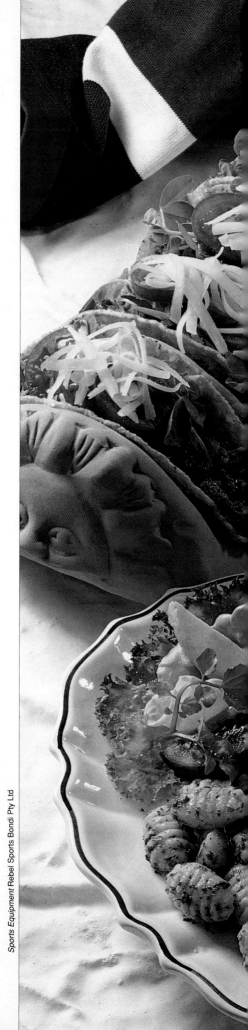

Sports Equipment Rebel Sports Bondi Pty Ltd

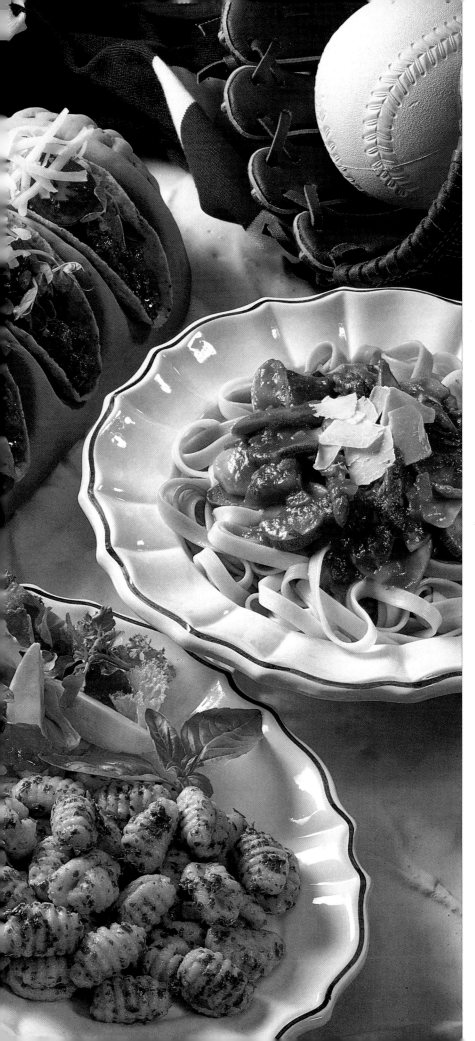

PASTA VEGETABLE MEDLEY

Serves 4

- ☐ **375 g (12 oz) spinach fettuccine**
- ☐ **375 g (12 oz) plain fettuccine**

VEGETABLE SAUCE
- ☐ **1 onion, finely chopped**
- ☐ **2 cloves garlic, crushed**
- ☐ **440 g (14 oz) canned peeled tomatoes, no-added-salt, undrained and mashed**
- ☐ **125 g (4 oz) creamed tomatoes, no-added-salt**
- ☐ **6 yellow baby squash or 3 courgettes, finely sliced**
- ☐ **150 g (5 oz) mangetout, trimmed**
- ☐ **250 g (8 oz) asparagus, cut into 4 cm (1¹/₂ in) lengths**
- ☐ **2 courgettes, chopped**
- ☐ **1 red pepper, chopped**
- ☐ **1 tablespoon chopped fresh basil**
- ☐ **30 g (1 oz) fresh Parmesan cheese, thinly sliced**

1 Cook pasta in a large saucepan of boiling water following packet directions. Drain and set aside to keep warm.

2 To make sauce, place onions, garlic and 1 tablespoon of juice from tomatoes in a large saucepan and cook for 3 minutes, or until onion is soft. Stir in tomatoes, creamed tomatoes, squash or courgettes, mangetout, asparagus, courgettes, red pepper and basil and cook for 4 minutes, or until vegetables are tender crisp.

Serving suggestion: Spoon sauce over hot pasta and top with slices of fresh Parmesan cheese.

560 Calories (2355 kilojoules) per serve
Carbohydrate	*97.0 g*	*High*
Protein	*27.0 g*	
Fat	*5.0 g*	*Low*
Fibre	*10.9 g*	*High*

VEGETABLE AND LENTIL SOUP

Serves 4

- ☐ 1 onion, finely chopped
- ☐ 1½ litres (2½ pt) vegetable stock
- ☐ 2 stalks celery, finely chopped
- ☐ 2 carrots, peeled and chopped
- ☐ 1 parsnip, peeled and chopped
- ☐ 2 courgettes, chopped
- ☐ 2 tomatoes, peeled, seeded and chopped
- ☐ 300 g (9½ oz) red lentils, cooked
- ☐ 1 tablespoon chopped fresh coriander
- ☐ freshly ground black pepper

1 Place onion and 2 tablespoons vegetable stock in a saucepan and cook for 3 minutes or until soft. Stir in celery, carrots, parsnip, courgettes and tomatoes, and cook for 2 minutes longer. Add remaining stock, bring to the boil, then reduce heat and simmer for 5-6 minutes.
2 Add lentils, coriander, and black pepper to taste and cook 4-5 minutes longer or until heated through.
Serving suggestion: Wholemeal bread and soup is a balanced and filling meal.

120 Calories (500 kilojoules) per serve
Carbohydrate	*20.0 g*	*High*
Protein	*8.0 g*	
Fat	*neg*	*Low*
Fibre	*6.7 g*	*High*

QUICK CURRY

Serves 4

- ☐ 2 teaspoons polyunsaturated oil
- ☐ 500 g (1 lb) lean lamb, trimmed of all visible fat and cut into strips
- ☐ 2 onions, cut into eighths
- ☐ 2 cloves garlic, crushed
- ☐ ½ small cauliflower, broken into florets
- ☐ 1 red pepper, cubed
- ☐ 1 tablespoon curry powder
- ☐ 1 teaspoon ground cumin
- ☐ 1 teaspoon ground turmeric
- ☐ 250 mL (8 fl oz) chicken stock
- ☐ 60 g (2 oz) frozen peas
- ☐ 3 tablespoons sultanas
- ☐ 2 teaspoons cornflour blended with
- ☐ 2 tablespoons water
- ☐ 200 g (6½ oz) low-fat natural yogurt
- ☐ 1 teaspoon garam marsala

1 Heat oil in a large frying pan or wok and stir-fry lamb for 3-4 minutes or until meat just changes colour. Remove from pan and set aside.
2 Place onions, garlic, cauliflower, red pepper, curry powder, cumin and turmeric in pan and cook for 5 minutes or until onion softens. Return lamb to pan. Stir in stock, peas and sultanas, then whisk in cornflour mixture and cook until curry boils and thickens. Stir in yogurt and garam marsala and heat gently without boiling.
Serving suggestion: Accompany curry with steamed rice.

325 Calories (1360 kilojoules per serve
Carbohydrate	*17.0 g*	*Low*
Protein	*33.0 g*	
Fat	*14.0 g*	*High*
Fibre	*4.2 g*	*Medium*

VEGETABLE PILAF

Serves 4

- ☐ 2 teaspoons polyunsaturated oil
- ☐ 2 red onions, sliced
- ☐ 1 clove garlic, crushed
- ☐ 250 g (8 oz) baby squash or courgettes, sliced
- ☐ 300 g (9½ oz) broccoli, cut into florets
- ☐ 300 g (9½ oz) cauliflower, cut into florets
- ☐ 200 g (6½ oz) button mushrooms, cut into quarters
- ☐ 1 red pepper, chopped
- ☐ 410 g (13 oz) brown rice, cooked

1 Heat oil in a large frying pan and cook onions and garlic for 3 minutes, or until onion is soft. Add baby squash or courgettes, broccoli, cauliflower, mushrooms and red pepper and cook for 4-5 minutes, or until vegetables are tender crisp.
2 Stir in rice and cook for 5 minutes longer or until rice is heated through.
Serving suggestion: Accompany with a mixed bean and crisp green salad.

225 Calories (950 kilojoules) per serve
Carbohydrate	*35.0 g*	*High*
Protein	*12.5 g*	
Fat	*4.0 g*	*Low*
Fibre	*8.9 g*	*High*

SUGARS

For some years athletes, particularly endurance athletes, were advised to avoid taking sugar immediately before exercise as it may drop blood sugar levels after exercise begins (theoretically because sugar stimulates the release of the hormone insulin whose job it is to decrease the level of sugar in the blood). Recent research indicates that whilst sugars can fall, in most cases the effect is transient and does not appear to affect performance. On the other hand, taking sugar immediately before exercise is not thought to benefit performance. Large quantities of concentrated sugar solutions may cause gastric upsets in some individuals.

Sugar on food labels refers to sucrose or table sugar. Other sugars or sweeteners such as fructose (fruit sugar), lactose (milk sugar), glucose, maltose, sorbitol, honey, etc. can be added to sweeten foods. Gram for gram, these sweeteners have a similar calorie/kilojoule value to sugar. Labels of products can legally state 'no added sugar' providing there is no added sucrose! If you are watching your sugar or calorie/kilojoule intake, look on the label for sugars 'incognito'. By contrast, saccharine, cyclamate and Nutrasweet have negligible calories/kilojoules.

Vegetable Pilaf, Vegetable and Lentil Soup, Quick Curry

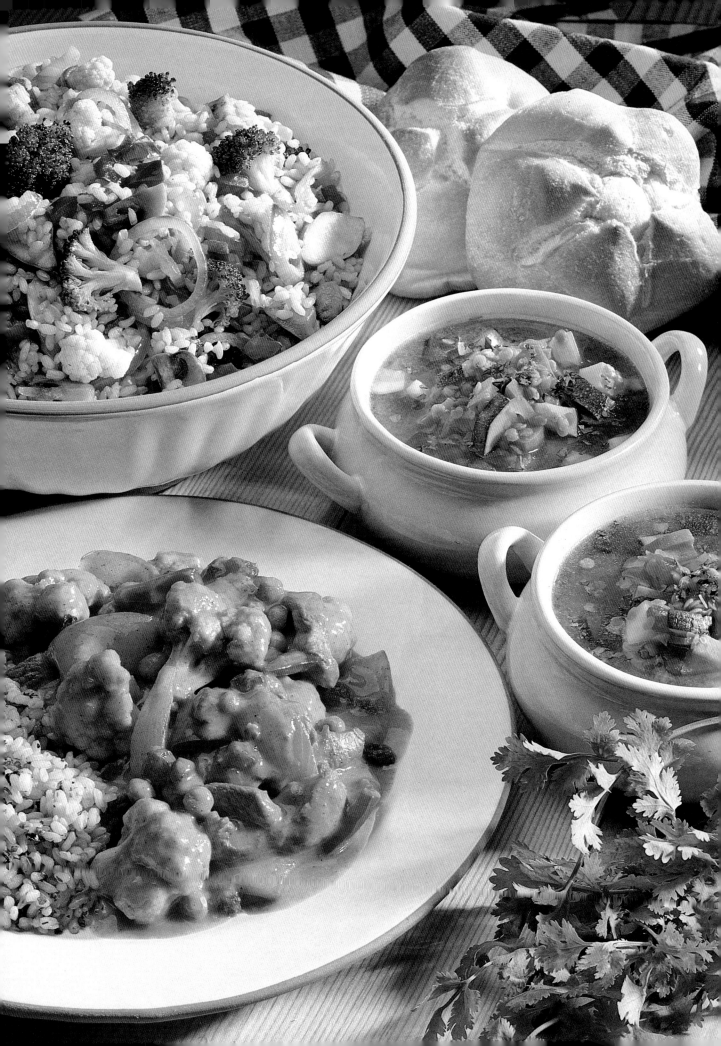

CHICKEN STIR-FRY

Serves 4

- ☐ 500 g (1 lb) chicken breast fillets, thinly sliced
- ☐ 1 red pepper, sliced
- ☐ 350 g (11 oz) broccoli, broken into florets
- ☐ 2 small courgettes, chopped
- ☐ 1 carrot, chopped
- ☐ 2 teaspoons cornflour blended with 1 tablespoon water
- ☐ 2 teaspoons grated fresh ginger
- ☐ 1 tablespoon honey
- ☐ 2 tablespoons soy sauce
- ☐ 1 tablespoon chilli sauce
- ☐ 1 tablespoon hoisin sauce

1   Heat a nonstick frying pan and cook chicken for 3-4 minutes or until tender. Remove from pan and set aside.

2   Add red pepper, broccoli, courgettes and carrot to pan and stir-fry for 2-3 minutes.

3   Stir in cornflour mixture, ginger, honey, soy sauce, chilli sauce and hoisin sauce and cook over a medium heat for 2-3 minutes or until sauce boils and thickens.

4   Return chicken to pan and stir-fry for 2-3 minutes longer or until heated through.

Serving suggestion: Delicious served on a bed of rice or noodles.

215 Calories (905 kilojoules) per serve

Carbohydrate	*12.0 g*	*Low*
Protein	*34.0 g*	
Fat	*3.5 g*	*Low*
Fibre	*5.2 g*	*Medium*

QUICK CUTLET CRUMBLE

Serves 4

- ☐ 4 x 200 g (6¹/₂ oz) white fish cutlets
- ☐ 2 tablespoons lime juice

HERB TOPPING
- ☐ 125 g (4 oz) wholemeal breadcrumbs, made from stale bread
- ☐ 45 g (1¹/₂ oz) instant rolled oats
- ☐ 2 tablespoons finely chopped fresh coriander
- ☐ 2 tablespoons finely snipped fresh chives
- ☐ 2 teaspoons olive oil
- ☐ 1 tablespoon vinegar
- ☐ freshly ground black pepper

1   Brush fish cutlets with lime juice and grill for 5 minutes on one side.

2   To make topping, place breadcrumbs, oats, coriander, chives, oil, vinegar and black pepper to taste in a bowl and mix to combine.

3   Turn fish and top each cutlet with topping and grill for 5 minutes, or until cooked through and topping is golden.

Serving suggestion: Garnish with lemon and accompany with new potatoes and a green salad.

325 Calories (1360 kilojoules) per serve

Carbohydrate	*20.0 g*	*Low*
Protein	*40.0 g*	
Fat	*9.0 g*	*Medium*
Fibre	*2.9 g*	*Medium*

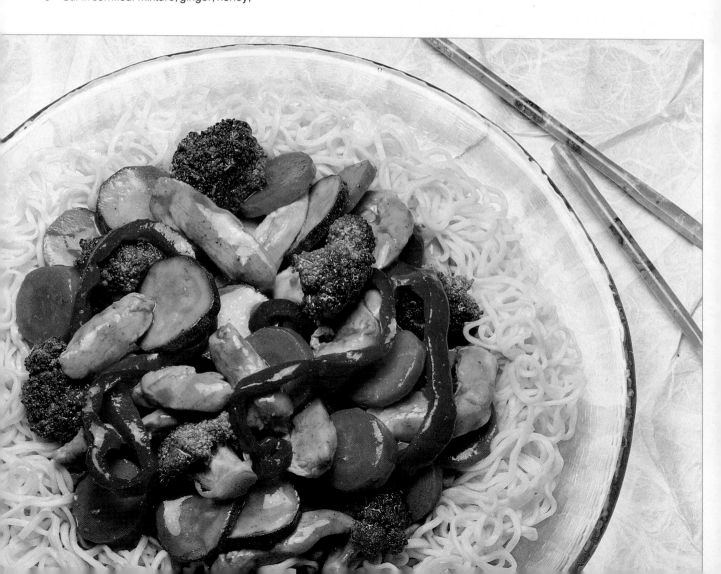

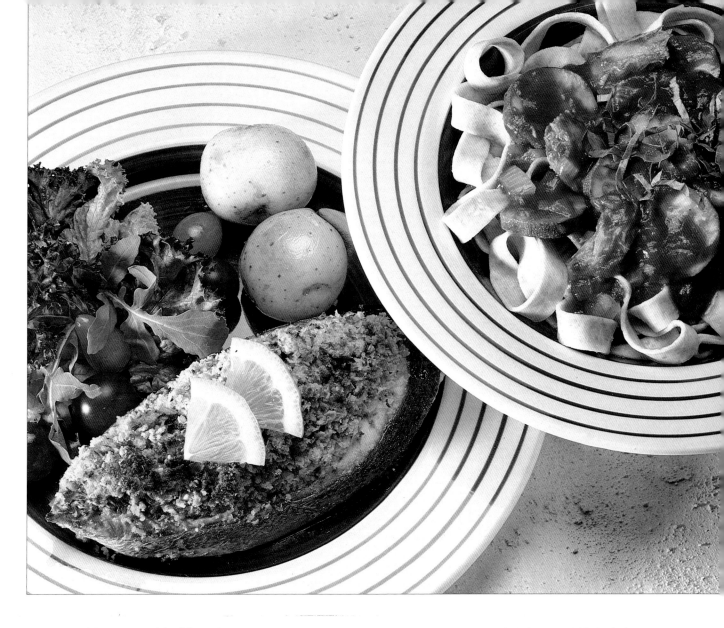

TAGLIATELLE WITH TUNA

Serves 4

- ☐ **375 g (12 oz) dried wholemeal tagliatelle or spaghetti**

TUNA SAUCE
- ☐ **1 onion, finely chopped**
- ☐ **1 clove garlic, crushed**
- ☐ **440 g (14 oz) canned peeled tomatoes, no-added-salt, undrained and mashed**
- ☐ **1 tablespoon tomato puree, no-added-salt**
- ☐ **1 tablespoon dry red wine**
- ☐ **2 courgettes, sliced**
- ☐ **440 g (14 oz) canned tuna in water, no-added-salt, drained and flaked**
- ☐ **1 tablespoon finely shredded fresh basil**

1 Cook pasta in a large saucepan of boiling water following packet directions. Drain and set aside to keep warm.

2 To make sauce, heat a nonstick frying pan and cook onion, garlic and 1 tablespoon of juice from tomatoes for 4-5 minutes, or until onion is soft. Stir in tomatoes, tomato puree, wine and courgettes and cook over a low heat for 5 minutes.

3 Add tuna and basil to pan and cook gently until heated through.

Serving suggestion: Place pasta on serving plates, spoon sauce over and garnish with basil. Serve with a mixed lettuce and herb salad and crusty bread.

To microwave: To make Tuna Sauce in the microwave, place onion and garlic in a microwave-safe dish and cook on HIGH (100%) for 2 minutes. Stir in tomatoes, passata, wine and courgettes and cook on HIGH (100%) for 3-4 minutes longer. Add tuna and basil and cook on HIGH (100%) for 3-4 minutes, longer.

375 Calories (1575 kilojoules) per serve

Carbohydrate	*48.0 g*	*Medium*
Protein	*35.0 g*	
Fat	*4.0 g*	*Low*
Fibre	*4.1 g*	*Medium*

Left: Chicken Stir-Fry
Above: Quick Cutlet Crumble,
Tagliatelle with Tuna

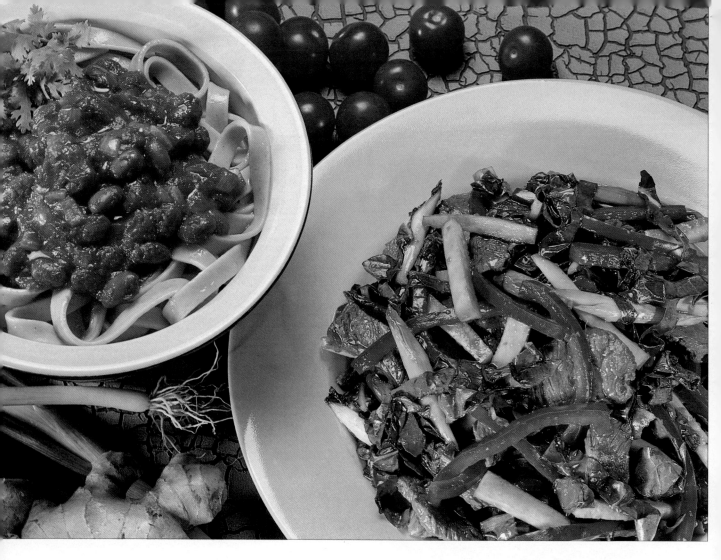

Mexican Chilli Pasta, Honey Beef

HONEY BEEF

Serves 4

- ☐ **1 tablespoon polyunsaturated oil**
- ☐ **500 g (1 lb) lean rump or topside steak, cut into thin strips**
- ☐ **1 red pepper, cut into thin strips**
- ☐ **4 spinach leaves, shredded**
- ☐ **3 spring onions, cut into 2.5 cm (1 in) diagonal lengths**
- ☐ **1 parsnip, peeled and cut into thin strips**
- ☐ **1 clove garlic, crushed**
- ☐ **2 teaspoons grated fresh ginger**
- ☐ **4 tablespoons soy sauce**
- ☐ **2 teaspoons honey**
- ☐ **2 teaspoons cornflour blended with 2 tablespoons dry sherry**

1   Heat 2 teaspoons oil in a frying pan or wok. Add meat, red pepper, spinach, spring onions and parsnip, and stir-fry for 2-3 minutes, or until meat changes colour. Remove mixture from pan and set aside.
2   Heat remaining oil and stir-fry garlic and ginger for 1-2 minutes. Return beef mixture to the pan. Combine soy sauce, honey and cornflour mixture, pour into pan and cook for 1-2 minutes longer or until heated through. Serve immediately.

280 Calories (1180 kilojoules) per serve

Carbohydrate	*9.0 g*	*Low*
Protein	*30.0 g*	
Fat	*13.0 g*	*High*
Fibre	*1.4 g*	*Low*

MEXICAN CHILLI PASTA

Serves 4

- ☐ **750 g (1¹/₂ lb) tomato or spinach fettuccine**

MEXICAN CHILLI SAUCE
- ☐ **2 onions, chopped**
- ☐ **1 clove garlic, crushed**
- ☐ **2 red chillies, finely chopped**
- ☐ **1 tablespoon water**
- ☐ **440 mL (14 fl oz) canned creamed tomatoes, no-added-salt**
- ☐ **440 g (14 oz) canned red kidney beans, drained**

1   Cook fettuccine in boiling water in a large saucepan following packet directions, drain and set aside to keep warm.
2   To make sauce, cook onion, garlic, chilli and water in large saucepan for 3-4 minutes, or until onion is soft. Stir in tomato puree and red kidney beans, bring to the boil, then reduce heat and simmer for 4-5 minutes, or until sauce thickens.
Serving suggestion: Spoon sauce over pasta.

605 Calories (2540 kilojoules) per serve

Carbohydrate	*109.0 g*	*High*
Protein	*35.0 g*	
Fat	*3.0 g*	*Low*
Fibre	*17.7 g*	*High*

Travellers' tales

Since the food supplied at sports venues is not designed to be healthy, competitors need to be prepared.

LOCAL EVENTS

● Take suitable foods with you.
● Packaged foods such as breads, cereals, juices or fruits (fresh, dried or canned) travel well.
● Commercially available sports drinks are a convenient snack and are a great back up.
● Take plain water to unfamiliar venues. Many sporting venues do not provide bubblers or water coolers for competitors.
● For large teams, special meals at restaurants and hotels can be organised. The team will not only eat better but, in general, more quickly!
● When competitors are away for several days consider the cooking facilities, food or menu that is available. Thinking ahead saves time and ensures competitors eat well.
● If staying at a hotel, stock the refrigerator with essentials such as cereals, juices, fruits, bread and milk.

OVERSEAS

The suggestions for competing at local events, with a few moderations, can be applied to overseas travel.
● Write out an itinerary of the countries to be visited and do a little research as to the types of foods likely to be available, safety of the water supply in the area, cost of food (so it can be included in your travel budget), and customs regulations regarding taking special sports drinks with you.
● The large variety and amount of food offered in athlete villages can be a temptation for many people. Aim to keep to your usual routine.

EATING IN UNFAMILIAR PLACES

Use the following checklist to help prevent illness:
● Use boiled, sterilised or bottled water. If the water supply is unsafe to drink, remember to avoid ice also!
● If bottled water is not available, canned or bottled soft drinks are preferable to the local water supply.
● If the water supply is unsafe, avoid anything raw which may be washed in water.
● Avoid all unpasteurised dairy products. If in doubt about pasteurisation, use long-life or powdered milk (made with sterile water).
● Watch how the food is handled. If you are in doubt about the hygiene, behind the scenes is likely to be worse! Eat at another venue.

TRAVELLERS' DIARRHOEA

One of the dangers of overseas travel is gastroenteritis, or so-called travellers' diarrhoea, symptoms for which include loose/frequent bowel motions, stomach cramps, nausea, vomiting and possibly fever. It has been estimated that travellers' diarrhoea affects between 30-60 per cent of athletes who travel overseas. Aside from the discomfort, the physical and psychological effects can be devastating and may prevent athletes from competing at all. Preventing the problem revolves around choosing food and fluids from hygienic outlets. The local water supply may also need to be avoided.

8 ways to prevent jetlag

● Do some light exercise before the flight.
● Request a seat in the nonsmoking section.
● Keep to 'home' time during the flight.
● Adjust to the new time schedule when you arrive.
● Drink liberal amounts of water.
● Stand up and stretch your legs on long flights.
● Avoid excess coffee, tea, cola drinks or alcohol.
● Eat moderately.

Time for a treat

STRAWBERRY AND PASSION FRUIT CHEESECAKE

Serves 6

- [ ] 100 g (3¹/₂ oz) wheatmeal biscuit crumbs
- [ ] 30 g (1 oz) polyunsaturated margarine, melted
- [ ] 2 teaspoons water

STRAWBERRY FILLING
- [ ] 2 x 135 g (4¹/₂ oz) tablets raspberry jelly
- [ ] 1 tablespoon gelatine
- [ ] 250 mL (8 fl oz) boiling water
- [ ] 170 g (5¹/₂ oz) low-fat natural yogurt
- [ ] 250 g (8 oz) low-fat cottage cheese
- [ ] pulp of 3 passion fruit
- [ ] 250 g (8 oz) strawberries, hulled and halved

1 Combine biscuit crumbs, margarine and water in a bowl. Press over base of a lightly greased 20 cm (8 in) springform tin. Refrigerate until firm.
2 Dissolve jelly and gelatine in water and set aside to cool, to room temperature. Place yogurt and cottage cheese in a food processor or blender and process until smooth. Add jelly mixture and process until combined. Stir in passion fruit pulp. Pour mixture over base and refrigerate until almost set. Arrange strawberries over top of cheesecake and return to refrigerator to set completely.

220 Calories (925 kilojoules) per serve

Carbohydrate	25.0 g	Low
Protein	12.0 g	
Fat	8.0 g	Medium
Fibre	3.4 g	Medium

HOT FRUIT SALAD

Serves 4

- [ ] 250 g (8 oz) dried fruit salad mix
- [ ] 90 g (3 oz) dried fruit medley
- [ ] 250 mL (8 fl oz) apricot nectar or orange juice
- [ ] 3 tablespoons lemon juice
- [ ] 3 tablespoons brandy
- [ ] 2 teaspoons honey, warmed
- [ ] 1 apple, chopped
- [ ] 250 g (8 oz) strawberries, hulled
- [ ] 250 g (8 oz) grapes or melon pieces
- [ ] 1 kiwi fruit, peeled and sliced
- [ ] 4 tablespoons low-fat natural yogurt

Place fruit salad, fruit medley, apricot nectar or orange juice, lemon juice, brandy and honey in a saucepan. Bring to the boil, then reduce heat and simmer for 10 minutes. Add apple, strawberries, grapes or melon, and kiwi fruit.

Serving suggestion: Serve hot or chilled with low-fat yogurt.

365 Calories (1540 kilojoules) per serve

Carbohydrate	83.0 g	High
Protein	6.0 g	
Fat	1.0 g	Low
Fibre	9.2 g	High

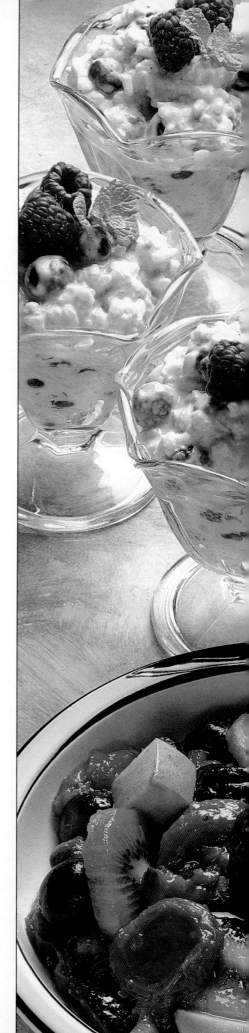

Strawberry and Passion Fruit Cheesecake, Hot Fruit Salad, Creamy Berry Rice

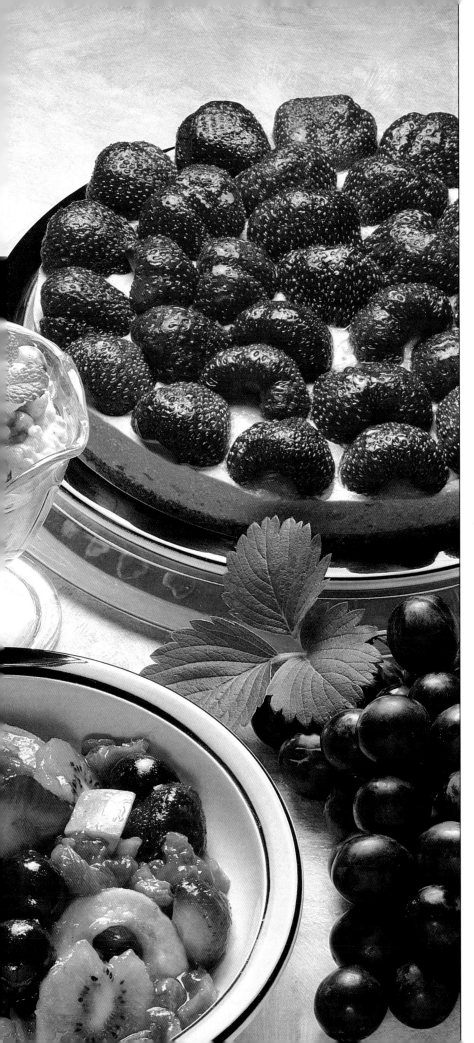

CREAMY BERRY RICE

Serves 4

- [ ] **100 g (3¹/₂ oz) short grain rice**
- [ ] **125 g (4 oz) blueberries or black currants**
- [ ] **125 g (4 oz) raspberries**
- [ ] **4 tablespoons low-fat natural yogurt**
- [ ] **3 tablespoons low-fat berry-flavoured yogurt**
- [ ] **185 mL (6 fl oz) evaporated skimmed milk**
- [ ] **1 tablespoon honey**
- [ ] **¹/₂ teaspoon ground mixed spice**

1 Cook rice in boiling water in a large saucepan of boiling water for 10-12 minutes, or until tender. Drain and rinse under cold running water.

2 Combine rice, blueberries, raspberries, natural and berry yogurt, evaporated milk, honey and mixed spice. Spoon into 4 individual serving dishes and chill.

Variation: You might like to use chopped, drained, canned fruits such as peaches, pears or apricots in place of the berries, and a complementary flavoured fruit yogurt in place of the berry yogurt.

260 Calories (1090 kilojoules) per serve

Carbohydrate	*50.0 g*	*High*
Protein	*13.0 g*	
Fat	*1.0 g*	*Low*
Fibre	*3.9 g*	*Medium*

ORANGE CREME CARAMELS

Serves 6
Oven temperature 180°C, 350°F, Gas 4

CARAMEL
- [ ] **125 mL (4 fl oz) water**
- [ ] **125 g (4 oz) sugar**

ORANGE CUSTARD
- [ ] **4 eggs, lightly beaten**
- [ ] **1 teaspoon vanilla essence**
- [ ] **3 tablespoons caster sugar**
- [ ] **60 g (2 oz) skimmed milk powder, sifted**
- [ ] **500 mL (16 fl oz) skimmed milk, scalded**
- [ ] **1 tablespoon grated orange rind**

1 To make Caramel, combine water and sugar in a small, heavy-based saucepan and cook, over a low heat, stirring constantly until sugar dissolves. Bring to the boil and boil, without stirring, until mixture turns a light golden brown. Pour into six individual lightly greased 125 mL (4 fl oz) capacity ramekins.

2 To make custard, place eggs, vanilla essence, sugar and skimmed milk powder in a mixing bowl and beat until sugar dissolves. Whisk in skimmed milk and orange rind, then pour into ramekins.

3 Place ramekins in a baking pan with enough boiling water to come halfway up sides of ramekins and bake for 20 minutes, or until a knife inserted into the centre of custard comes out clean.

4 Remove ramekins from baking pan and set aside to cool. Chill.

Serving suggestion: Invert chilled desserts onto serving plates and accompany with canned or stewed apricots.

225 Calories (940 kilojoules) per serve

Carbohydrate	*39.0 g*	*High*
Protein	*9.0 g*	
Fat	*4.0 g*	*Low*
Fibre	*neg*	*Low*

FRUITY STRUDEL

Serves 4
Oven temperature 200°C, 400°F, Gas 6

- [ ] **5 sheets filo pastry**
- [ ] **15 g (¹/₂ oz) polyunsaturated margarine, melted**

FILLING
- [ ] **1 apple, peeled and chopped**
- [ ] **2 pears, peeled and chopped**
- [ ] **125 g (4 oz) mixed dried fruit**
- [ ] **60 g (2 oz) wholemeal breadcrumbs, made from stale bread**
- [ ] **3 tablespoons caster sugar**
- [ ] **¹/₂ teaspoon ground cinnamon**
- [ ] **1 teaspoon grated lemon rind**
- [ ] **2 tablespoons orange juice**
- [ ] **2 teaspoons sugar**

1 To make filling, combine apple, pears, dried fruit, breadcrumbs, caster sugar, cinnamon, lemon rind and orange juice in saucepan. Bring to the boil, then reduce heat and simmer, covered, for 10 minutes or until mixture thickens. Remove from heat and set aside to cool.

2 Layer pastry sheets, brushing every second layer with margarine. Spoon filling diagonally across one edge of pastry sheets. Roll up strudel, turning in sides as you roll. Place on a lightly greased baking tray. Brush top with a little margarine and sprinkle with sugar. Bake for 10-15 minutes, or until golden brown.

320 Calories (1350 kilojoules) per serve

Carbohydrate	*67.5 g*	*High*
Protein	*5.0 g*	
Fat	*4.0 g*	*Low*
Fibre	*5.9 g*	*Medium*

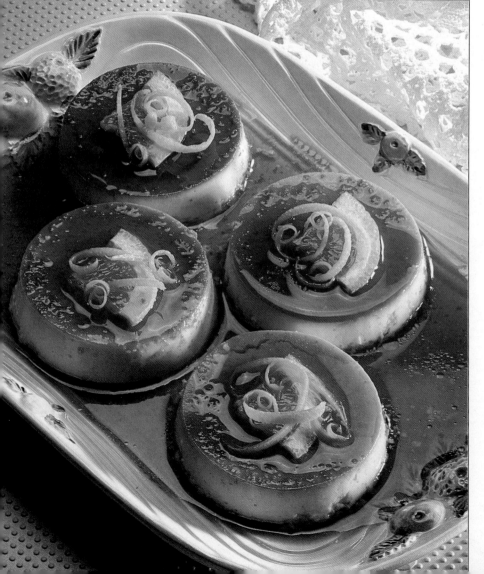

Left: Orange Creme Caramels
Right: Fruity Strudel, Apricot Bread Pudding

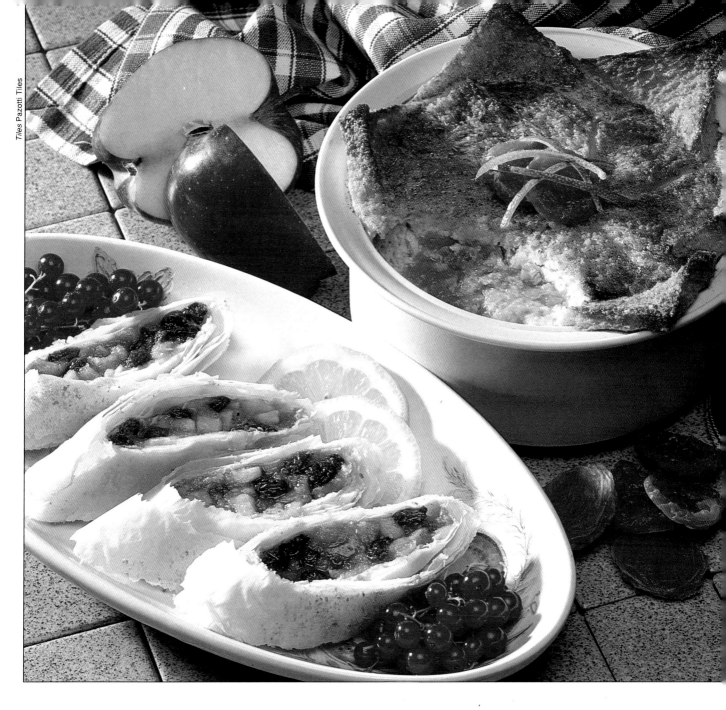

APRICOT BREAD PUDDING

Serves 4
Oven temperature 180°C, 350°F, Gas 4

☐ **10 slices wholemeal bread, crusts removed**
☐ **75 g (2¹/₂ oz) chopped dried apricots**
☐ **200 g (6¹/₂ oz) yolk-free egg mix, thawed**
☐ **2 tablespoons honey**
☐ **250 mL (8 fl oz) evaporated skimmed milk**
☐ **500 mL (16 fl oz) skimmed milk**
☐ **¹/₂ teaspoon ground cinnamon**

1 Cut each slice of bread in half diagonally. Arrange a third of the bread triangles in a lightly greased 20 cm (8 in) souffle dish. Sprinkle with half the apricots and layer with another third of bread triangles. Top with remaining apricots and bread, placing 6 triangles around the outside of the dish and covering the pudding with remaining slices.

2 Combine egg mix, honey, evaporated skimmed milk and skimmed milk. Pour over bread then sprinkle with cinnamon.

3 Place souffle dish in a baking pan with enough boiling water to come halfway up the sides of the dish and bake for 40 minutes, or until a knife inserted into the centre of pudding comes out clean.

385 Calories (1605 kilojoules) per serve

Carbohydrate	54.5 g	Medium
Protein	23.0 g	
Fat	8.5 g	Low
Fibre	6.8 g	High

YOLK-FREE EGG MIX

Yolk-free egg mix is a low cholesterol mix and is available as a frozen product from supermarkets. It is made from egg whites, polyunsaturated vegetable oil and skimmed milk and can be used in cooking in place of whole eggs. One sachet (100 g/3¹/₂ oz) is the equivalent of two whole eggs. Try using this mix in recipes in place of eggs.

SUMMER PUDDING

Serves 4

- [ ] **250 g (8 oz) blueberries**
- [ ] **3 tablespoons brown sugar**
- [ ] **4 tablespoons blackcurrant juice**
- [ ] **200 g (6¹/₂ oz) raspberries**
- [ ] **250 g (8 oz) strawberries, hulled**
- [ ] **440 g (14 oz) canned stoneless cherries, drained**
- [ ] **10 slices wholemeal bread, crusts removed**

1   Place blueberries or black currants, brown sugar and blackcurrant juice in large saucepan and cook over a low heat for 5-10 minutes, or until berries are tender. Add raspberries, strawberries and cherries and set aside to cool.

2   Line a 1 litre (1³/₄ pt) pudding basin with bread. Spoon half the cooled fruit mixture into basin and top with a layer of bread. Add remaining fruit and finish with a final layer of bread. Pour over any remaining liquid.

3   Place a saucer small enough to fit inside the basin on top of pudding and weigh it down with a 500 g (1 lb) weight (a can of fruit or bowl of water is ideal). Refrigerate overnight.

Serving suggestion: Turn onto a serving plate and cut into wedges.

To microwave: Place blueberries, brown sugar and blackcurrant juice in a microwave dish and cook on high for 3-4 minutes. Complete as above.

310 Calories (1290 kilojoules) per serve

Carbohydrate	64.0 g	High
Protein	9.0 g	
Fat	2.0 g	Low
Fibre	13.0 g	High

PEACHY CRUNCHY CRUMBLE

Serves 4
Oven temperature 180°C, 350°F, Gas 4

- [ ] **2 x 440 g (14 oz) canned peach halves, drained and liquid reserved**
- [ ] **pulp of 2 passion fruit**
- [ ] **90 g (3 oz) untoasted muesli**
- [ ] **2 tablespoons plain flour**
- [ ] **1 tablespoon brown sugar**
- [ ] **30 g (1 oz) polyunsaturated margarine**
- [ ] **4 tablespoons chopped walnuts**
- [ ] **1 teaspoon ground cinnamon**

1   Pour reserved peach liquid into a shallow ovenproof dish. Then arrange peach halves cavity side up in dish. Spoon a little passion fruit pulp into each cavity.

2   Combine muesli, flour and sugar. Rub in margarine, then stir in walnuts and cinnamon. Sprinkle mixture over peaches and bake for 20 minutes.

Serving suggestion: Serve with low-fat natural or fruit-flavoured yogurt.

345 Calories (1450 kilojoules) per serve

Carbohydrate	49.0 g	Medium
Protein	6.0 g	
Fat	14.0 g	Medium
Fibre	7.4 g	High

TROPICAL CREPES

Serves 4

- [ ] **125 g (4 oz) plain flour, sifted**
- [ ] **2 eggs, lightly beaten**
- [ ] **250 mL (8 fl oz) skimmed milk**

FILLING
- [ ] **200 g (6¹/₂ oz) reduced-fat ricotta cheese**
- [ ] **1 tablespoon honey**
- [ ] **3 tablespoons flaked almonds, toasted**
- [ ] **1 mango, peeled and thinly sliced**
- [ ] **220 g (7 oz) canned pineapple pieces, drained**
- [ ] **shredded coconut, toasted**

1   Place flour in a bowl. Combine eggs and milk and stir in flour a little at a time until mixture is smooth. Set aside for 30 minutes. Pour 3 tablespoons of mixture into a heated nonstick frying pan and cook over a medium heat until golden brown on each side. Remove from pan and set aside to keep warm. Repeat with remaining mixture.

2   To make filling, combine ricotta cheese, honey and almonds in a small bowl and mix well. Place spoonfuls of ricotta mixture over one half of each crepe. Top with slices of mango and pineapple pieces, then fold crepes into triangles.

Serving suggestion: Sprinkle with shredded coconut and serve immediately.

Variation: Any fruit can be used in place of the mango and pineapple. You might like to use fresh berries, canned or fresh apricots, peaches or pears.

Do ahead: Cook crepes and allow to cool. Stack crepes, interleaved with plastic food wrap and place in a freezer bag and freeze for up to 3 months. Reheat frozen crepes in the microwave for 20 seconds per crepe, or until just warm. Fill and serve.

370 Calories (1555 kilojoules) per serve

Carbohydrate	45.0 g	Low
Protein	17.0 g	
Fat	13.0 g	Medium
Fibre	4.1 g	Medium

NUTRITION TIPS

● Fresh fruit and vegetables subjected to the environment after picking lose vitamins. The amount lost depends on handling and how long before they are consumed. Snap-frozen vegetables escape excessive environmental exposure and often have a higher content of vitamins than those bought from the grocer. Although vitamins are inevitably lost with food handling and processing, a varied and well balanced diet will provide plenty of vitamins.

● Butter and margarine provide the same kilojoules (calories). The major difference between them is the type of fat they contain, butter being saturated, margarine predominantly poly-unsaturated. If small quantities of either are consumed it makes little difference which one is chosen. People with a high blood cholesterol level are advised to replace butter with polyunsaturated margarine, as a way of decreasing their saturated fat intake.

● Honey and sugar (brown, white or raw) are both simple carbohydrates that provide energy (kilojoules/ calories), yet insignificant amounts of vitamins or minerals. There is no health benefit in substituting honey, brown or raw sugar for white sugar.

Summer Pudding, Peachy Crunchy Crumble, Tropical Crepes

THE WOULD-BE-IF-THEY-COULD-BE VITAMINS…BUT THEY AREN'T

Supplements other than vitamins are often used by active people, either to improve performance or health. The proposed use of these and the scientific basis – or lack of it – is outlined in the following table.

SUBSTANCE	PROPOSED USE AND CLAIMS (not necessarily proven)	COMMENTS ON CLAIMS
Aloe vera	Alternative treatment for: burns, arthritis, infection, diabetes, multiple sclerosis, cancer	Claims are anecdotal. No benefits proven scientifically.
Amino acids	Increases muscle bulk.	More research needed. Current evidence does not support claims in doses taken (see page 37).
Bee pollen	Improves athletic ability.	Contains some essential nutrients but quantities are too small to be significant. Potentially allergenic.
Brewer's yeast	Improves athletic ability.	Good source of B vitamins. High in the minerals chromium and selenium. High in purines so is unsuitable for anyone with gout. Claims for athletic performance not scientifically proven.
Co-enzyme Q	Improves athletic performance.	Limited research does not support claims.
Garlic	Athletes foot, anti-ageing, respiratory ailments.	May decrease blood fats. Other claims not proven scientifically.
Ginseng	Fertility, aphrodisiac, relieves fatigue, stress, reduces blood fats.	In large doses may cause insomnia and depression. Other claims not proven scientifically.
Inosine	Improves athletic performance.	Limited research does not support claims.
Kelp	Iodine supplement to improve thyroid function.	Does contain iodine and vitamin B12. Also contains arsenic!
Pangamic acid (Vitamin B15)	Improves athletic performance.	Not a true vitamin. Sold as a whole range of compounds, some contain substances which are potentially cancer causing. Scientific research has found no performance benefits.
Royal jelly	Improves athletic performance.	Contains pantothenic acid and pyridoxine (vitamin B6) but in quantities too small to be of nutritional importance – other than to bees for which the substance was intended. Claims are not proven scientifically.
Wheat germ	Improves physical performance.	Good source of fibre. Contains iron, zinc, vitamins E and B complex amongst others.

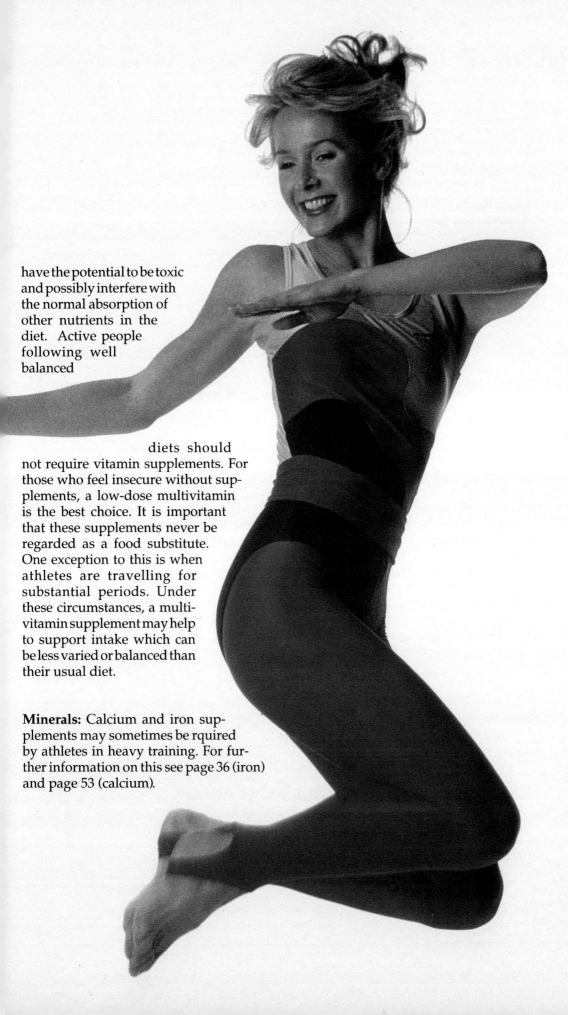

have the potential to be toxic and possibly interfere with the normal absorption of other nutrients in the diet. Active people following well balanced

diets should not require vitamin supplements. For those who feel insecure without supplements, a low-dose multivitamin is the best choice. It is important that these supplements never be regarded as a food substitute. One exception to this is when athletes are travelling for substantial periods. Under these circumstances, a multivitamin supplement may help to support intake which can be less varied or balanced than their usual diet.

Minerals: Calcium and iron supplements may sometimes be rquired by athletes in heavy training. For further information on this see page 36 (iron) and page 53 (calcium).

JANEART LTD/THE IMAGE BANK

Be healthy and slim

A major proportion of the weight-loss diets promoted to the public are based on 'fads' and have no scientific basis.

The following checklist will help you to judge whether your diet is a sensible one.

DIETERS' CHECKLIST

● The diet should include a variety of foods like bread and cereals, fruits and vegetables, lean meat and alternatives (eggs, poultry, seafood and legumes), dairy foods and limited amounts of fats and oils. Some food from each food group needs to be included daily.

● The diet needs to include regular meals that will fit into your lifestyle.

● The energy level should not be less than 1000 calories (4200 kilojoules) per day. Active people rarely need diets less than 1500 calories (6300 kilojoules) per day.

● The diet should allow for a gradual weight loss of 0.5-1 kg (1-2 lb) per week. Rapid weight reduction increases the loss of water and muscle. Weight loss in overweight children or adolescents needs to be managed carefully as growth may be compromised if losses are rapid. Weight maintenance or, at most, gradual weight loss is recommended. In this way they can 'grow out' of their excess weight.

● The diet should use regular foods and not include special supplements.

EATING DISORDERS

Looking slim is fashionable in our society and many people exercise specifically to achieve or maintain a slim body. For some, such as ballet dancers, gymnasts and figure skaters, slimness is also an aesthetic requirement. Even at the non-elite level there is often intense pressure to maintain a slim body. Some people participating in these sports have a metabolism and body type which lends itself to slimness. They seemingly have little difficulty in maintaining the right weight or shape. Others fight a constant battle to achieve what is sometimes an unrealistic weight for them.

Disordered eating, such as anorexia nervosa or bulimia, is closely associated with social pressures or personal desires to be slim. It is more common in young women than men.

While dieting for cosmetic or competitive reasons is a common feature of disordered eating, there may also be other underlying psychological problems. People with an eating disorder usually need to seek outside counselling – nutritional, psychological or a combination of both. Early diagnosis and treatment is often difficult as those affected generally deny they have the condition.

Athletes, coaches and parents need to be realistic about how appropriate a particular weight or body fat goal is and give due consideration to the physical and psychological dangers associated with the pressure of imposing to inflexible and unrealistic goals.

Anorexia nervosa is characterised by:
● An intense desire to be slim.
● Dramatic weight loss due to self starvation.
● In some cases excessive exercise.
● Normal amounts of food appear excessive.
● Every calorie (kilojoule) consumed is often counted.
● Menstruation may become irregular or stop all together.

Bulimia is characterised by:
● Periods of starvation as in anorexia.
● But these are broken by binges where large quantities of food are consumed.
● In some cases, self-induced vomiting, laxatives or diuretics are used.
● Bulimics are not typically underweight, they may be overweight or normal weight.

Useful information

In this book, ingredients such as fish and meat are given in grams (ounces) so you know how much to buy. It is handy to have:
● A small inexpensive set of kitchen scales.
Other ingredients in our recipes are given in spoons so you will need:
● A set of measuring spoons (1 tablespoon, 1 teaspoon, 1/2 teaspoon and 1/4 teaspoon).
● A transparent graduated measuring jug (1 litre or 250 mL) for measuring liquids.
● Spoon measures are level.

QUICK CONVERTER

Metric	Imperial
5 mm	1/4 in
1 cm	1/2 in
2 cm	3/4 in
2.5 cm	1 in
5 cm	2 in
10 cm	4 in
15 cm	6 in
20 cm	8 in
23 cm	9 in
25 cm	10 in
30 cm	12 in

MEASURING LIQUIDS

Metric	Imperial
30 mL	1 fl oz
60 mL	2 fl oz
90 mL	3 fl oz
125 mL	4 fl oz
155 mL	5 fl oz
170 mL	5 1/2 fl oz
185 mL	6 fl oz
220 mL	7 fl oz
250 mL	8 fl oz
500 mL	16 fl oz
600 mL	20 fl oz (1 pt)
750 mL	1 1/4 pt
1 litre	1 3/4 pt
1.2 litres	2 pt

METRIC CUPS & SPOONS

Metric	Imperial
60 mL	2 fl oz
80 mL	2 1/2 fl oz
125 mL	4 fl oz
250 mL	8 fl oz
Spoons	
1.25 mL	1/4 teaspoon
2.5 mL	1/2 teaspoon
5 mL	1 teaspoon
20 mL	1 tablespoon

MEASURING DRY INGREDIENTS

Metric	Imperial
15 g	1/2 oz
30 g	1 oz
60 g	2 oz
90 g	3 oz
125 g	4 oz
155 g	5 oz
185 g	6 oz
220 g	7 oz
250 g	8 oz
280 g	9 oz
315 g	10 oz
375 g	12 oz
410 g	13 oz
440 g	14 oz
470 g	15 oz
500 g	16 oz (1 lb)
750 g	1 lb 8 oz
1 kg	2 lb
1.5 kg	3 lb

OVEN TEMPERATURES

°C	°F	Gas Mark
120	250	1/2
140	275	1
150	300	2
160	325	3
180	350	4
190	375	5
200	400	6
220	425	7
240	475	8
250	500	9

Index

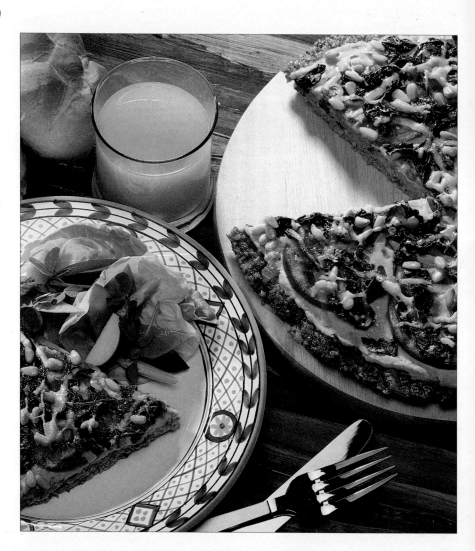

ACKNOWLEDGMENTS

The publishers wish to thank the following Admiral Appliances; Black & Decker (Australasia) Pty Ltd; Blanco Appliances; Knebel Kitchens; Leigh Mardon Pty Ltd; Master Foods of Australia; Meadow Lea Foods; Namco Cookware; Ricegrowers' Co-op Mills Ltd; Sunbeam Corporation Ltd; Tycraft Pty Ltd distributors of Braun, Australia; White Wings Foods for their assistance during recipe testing and photography.

Chris Gerranis (Physiotherapist) and Maria Kokkinakos (Dietitian Nutritionist) for their assistance during production.